Sexual Abuse and the Primary Care Doctor

PSYCHOSEXUAL MEDICINE SERIES

Edited by Ruth L. Skrine MB, ChB, MRCGP

Psychosexual Medicine is a discipline which uses a combined body and mind approach to problems related to sexuality, and which stresses the importance of the doctor–patient relationship. The method derives from psychoanalysis but is distinct in that the practitioner listens to unconscious material over a focused, narrow field. The work of many doctors and nurses and of some physiotherapists, provides opportunities for physical examination and treatment of the genital area which are unavailable to non-medical sexual therapists. Both physical and psychological problems and the interaction between them can be explored at the time of physical examination.

This series forms part of the developing body of knowledge held by members of the Institute of Psychosexual Medicine, formed in London in 1974. The books are for doctors and their colleagues who are interested in a psychosomatic approach to sexual problems particularly those working in general practice and gynaecology, as well as psychological and genito-urinary medicine.

Other titles in this series

Psychosexual Training and the Doctor/Patient Relationship
Edited by R. L. Skrine

Introduction to Psychosexual Medicine
Edited by R. L. Skrine

Sexual Abuse and the Primary Care Doctor

GILL WAKLEY

Principal in a general practice in North Staffordshire

CHAPMAN & HALL

London · New York · Tokyo · Melbourne · Madras

UK	Chapman & Hall, 2–6 Boundary Row, London SE1 8HN
USA	Chapman & Hall, 29 West 35th Street, New York NY 10001
JAPAN	Chapman & Hall Japan, Thomson Publishing Japan, Hirakawacho Nemoto Building, 7F, 1–7–11 Hirakawa-cho, Chiyoda-ku, Tokyo 102
AUSTRALIA	Chapman & Hall Australia, Thomas Nelson Australia, 102 Dodds Street, South Melbourne, Victoria 3205
INDIA	Chapman & Hall India, R. Seshadri, 32 Second Main Road, CIT East, Madras 600 035

First edition 1991

Typeset in Linotron Times 10½ on 11½pt by Intype, London

Printed in Great Britain by St. Edmundsbury Press, Bury St. Edmunds, Suffolk.

ISBN 0 412 415801

British Library Cataloguing in Publication Data
Wakley, G.M.
Sexual abuse and the primary care doctor.
I. Title
362.8

ISBN 0–412–41580–1

Library of Congress Cataloging-in-Publication Data
Available

Contents

Acknowledgements

I am greatly indebted to all the patients involved in these studies. They are the principal source of education for doctors and without the study of case presentations no progress in the understanding of this difficult subject could be made. Details from the case histories of some of the patients studied by doctors in seminars have been used to illustrate this book. Considerable efforts have been made to disguise any characteristics which might lead to a patient being identified, while attempting to preserve sufficient of the interactions between doctor and patient to give an accurate picture of the encounters described.

I must thank all the members of the seminars of which I have been a part, or have led, for increasing my understanding. Particularly I would like to thank those members of the Institute of Psychosexual Medicine who have provided me with stimulation for examination of new concepts, either from their case presentations, or their insights presented in the discussion of the cases: Dr H. Backer; Dr S. Buck; Dr J. Coombs; Dr K. Draper; Dr M. Gill; Dr J. Gilley; Dr F. Hutchinson; Dr T. Main; Dr A. Morgan; Dr J. Peebles; Dr A. Smith; Dr G. Tattersall; Dr R. Thexton; Dr A. Tobert; Dr B. Tully and Dr P. Tunnadine. However, the opinions and ideas in this book are my own, have been modified during writing, and will continue to change as understanding of sexual abuse progresses.

Last, but not least, I must thank Dr R. Skrine and Mr J. Matthews for encouraging me to try to write this book and for their unstinting help in the final stages.

Preface

The importance of identifying a history of sexual abuse is now well recognized by doctors who know that the problem may lie behind a presentation of physical illness, relationship problems, unhappiness or sexual and psychological difficulties. It is, however, impossible to say accurately how often sexual abuse is a factor, because in so many cases it is not acknowledged consciously, or is hidden away where it is inaccessible without skilled help.

The majority of the books on sexual abuse have been written from particular standpoints. There are now many such books for social workers who are called in because of revelations by children. Stories are written by those who have suffered in order to help themselves overcome their difficulties and help others to do the same. There are accounts of how to detect the signs of abuse for police surgeons, forensic psychiatrists or paediatricians which spell out the unpleasant and distressing nature of the work. There are examinations of the family interactions by family therapists, accounts of individual long-term psychotherapy with victims by adult or child psychotherapists and advice on group therapy methods for lay or professional workers. All of these deal with the problem after it has been exposed and after it has been referred for specialist help. There was no book, however, to illuminate the skills, attitudes and knowledge needed by the doctor (or nurse) of first contact.

General practitioners or family physicians are the most likely to be the doctor of first contact, but anyone who works in contact with patients may be involved. Many people feel that family planning clinics or contraceptive consultations are the right place to bring sexual problems and distress. Other sources of help such as youth advisory clinics or medical facilities in further education establishments may be viewed in the same way. Departments of genito-urinary medicine and other sources of help for sexually-transmitted diseases will be consulted directly and will be involved when exploitative sexual activity has exposed someone to infection. Psychiatric services, including the specialist psychosexual clinics, should be particularly aware of the problems produced by previous sexual abuse.

It is clear that specialists in all disciplines need to be conscious of the possibility that sexual abuse may be implicated in the aetiology of some complaints. The patient who presents to the plastic surgeon for remodelling of her body, the one pressing the surgeon to remove the 'badness' inside, the woman whose pelvic pain goes on being investigated by one gynaecologist after another; all need to have a doctor who is sensitive to what is not being said. Those who are responsible for seeing people with chronic illnesses (like rheumatologists or renal physicians) may elicit accounts of sexual abuse when they seek to help their patients come to terms with long-term illness and disability.

Consider the child who sees a surgeon for his tummy ache, a paediatrician for his eating problems, the child-guidance clinic for his school refusal, the urologist for his enuresis and the dermatologist for his eczema; at least one of the many professionals in contact with the child must consider the distress of the whole child and identify the underlying causes.

Health visitors, school nurses, district nurses, practice nurses and family planning nurses, all have their share of revelations by children or adults. The health professionals also need to be able to help the parents, the teachers, the police officers and others who may be the first recipient of the news.

This book makes a start on the attitudes, skills and knowledge necessary to enable professionals to cope with the experience of being the first to be told. In the first chapter the necessity of preparation for the moment of disclosure is discussed, the clues which help to suggest that sexual abuse has occurred are illustrated and the responsibility of the listener (who may be both first and last to hear the unburdening) is delineated. The second chapter looks at the anxieties of not knowing what is normal – where the boundaries between acceptable loving and unacceptable exploitation belong. The development of sensuality and the anxieties of parents are placed within the wider framework of social attitudes towards family organization.

Moving on from younger children and the anxieties of their parents, the turbulence of adolescence is examined. The special difficulties of the professional dealing with the 'not still a child but not yet an adult' and the confusions brought about by coping with both the teenager and the parent together are illustrated by case studies. The lack of attention and protection by the mother seems to be particularly important and may be a risk factor for future difficulties with relationships, sexuality and self-worth.

The theme of the mother who did not care is continued into Chapter 4 and is shown together with an illustration of the difficulties which occur when sexual abuse is presented and distracts attention from the real problem. The enigmas posed by the guilt, the excitement and the denial of sexual abuse are examined in the next chapter. These subjects are often as distressing for the listener as the informant, and it is difficult to resist the temptation to flee to other, safer, subjects.

Further hidden problems are discussed at greater length

in Chapter 6 and some common themes emerge, notably the concept of powerlessness of those abused, the power of patriarchal figures, the role of mothers and grandmothers and the cycle of powerlessness repeating the patterns in subsequent generations.This is followed by illustrations of how to cope with those patients damaged beyond repair and the necessity of limiting the caring that can be undertaken without damage to the doctor or to other patients.

In Chapter 8 the ways of dealing with current abuse are discussed. Careful procedures have been laid down, but the book looks beyond such procedures to the dilemmas faced by the general practitioner who has responsibility not just for the child, but also for the rest of the family. The effect of the disclosure on the individual doctor is explored, and comment is made on the ethical and technical issues involved; these cannot (and should not) be solved by doctors alone but need responses from society in general.

An account of sexual abuse would not be complete without a chapter on rape. The similarities between rape and sexual abuse in childhood are elucidated and some of the myths and misunderstandings exposed. The powerlessness of an abused child may persist to make the adult more vulnerable to attack or exploitation. Case histories illustrate ways of dealing with the emotional turmoil of sexual assault and releasing the anger identified in the doctor-patient relationship. Other people involved in the trauma of sexual abuse, the relatives of the abused and the abusers, professionals and others not directly involved, all need support and care from a doctor who does not appear to be overwhelmed by the story. The doctors who have to cope with their own emotional response will also need support; time for reflection and repair is essential to maintain the healthiness of those who care.

The last chapter looks at how people cope with their experience of sexual abuse, the essential knowledge that the doctor should have, the options for treatment, and the special requirements of the abused child. Doctors need to know their limitations – whether their expertise is sufficient and whether to avoid involvement because of their personal feelings and experiences.

More information is needed to help us to a better understanding of why and how sexual exploitation occurs. Our efforts at prevention can then become more focused and effective than the counter measures being employed now. The recent publicity about satanic rituals serves as a reminder that it is all too easy to forget that most abuse takes place in the security of the home by people who are well-known to the abused. It is much more comforting to believe that abusers are strange, bizarre individuals, not like us or our neighbours. Prevention cannot be vested in the few – the social worker, the probation officer, the designated paediatrician – but must become the responsibility of everyone. Adults and children must have the right to decide for themselves how their bodies are to be used; the vulnerable need extra protection. Where exploitation occurs, professionals must be ready to hear and take action when required.

Foreword

In recent years there has been considerable concentration by professionals upon the incidence of sexual abuse, the need for protection of children and prevention of abuse. There has been less emphasis upon the continuing problems of those who have been abused in the past and how the medical and allied professions should respond to those who call upon them for help. This interesting, thoughtful and thought-provoking book raises many of the problems which might arise for the medical profession and gives helpful and sensitive advice on the approach to meeting them.

As a layman I am conscious that I do not have either the training or the experience to make appropriate comments on any details of the book. But I am aware of the lack of knowledge and experience, and consequential anxiety, of many in the medical and wider fields when faced with coping with problems such as those illustrated in this book. The observations of the author with the examples should be helpful to a more varied audience than medical practitioners, and the book deserves a wider reading public.

It is, however, primarily to the medical practitioner that Dr Wakley targets her observations and she deals both with the child and with the adult who suffered as a child. The possibility of sexual abuse as one answer to various long-term and deep-seated problems suffered by adults is likely to be one which may not have been previously considered. Such a possibility can no longer be rejected out of hand. The personal prejudices of those who receive confidences need to be recognized; their reactions to a subject which may be for some upsetting, for others disagreeable, to some evoke other responses of which as professionals they should be aware. For all engaged in dealing with children or with adults suffering from childhood events, the stress of such work on the professionals ought not to be under-estimated or brushed aside. One particularly interesting comment was the role of the general practitioner, not only as the first call in primary care but also as an always available and continuous source of care for the patient.

Dr Wakley has filled a gap and provided a valuable addition to the study of the problems created by sexual abuse.

Elizabeth Butler-Sloss

1

The problem in primary care

Over the last few years doctors working in primary care have seen an increase in the number of people presenting with a history of sexual abuse. The commonest reactions from doctors are panic ('What am I supposed to do/say?') and denial ('This can't be true.'). Doctors feel ill-equipped to deal with this emotive problem because of lack of expertise, inadequate resources, and their own problems and difficulties in dealing with the emotions produced by hearing about abusive episodes.

Within the population of any one practice there are only a handful of children who are currently being, or have recently been, sexually abused. However, doctors see large numbers of patients whose lives are touched by the media's excitement with this topic. Some of these patients turn to the doctors in the hope that they can provide expert advice about what constitutes normal touching of a child by an adult. There are also a substantial number of patients who give a history of sexual abuse occurring in the past, and who turn to the doctor for help.

THE LIMITATIONS OF A SPECIALIST VIEW

Almost all the accounts of therapy for patients who have experienced sexual abuse in the past are written from specialist standpoints. Therapists who have been trained in particular disciplines tends to view their patients or clients in particular ways. Many of these seem too rigid to be applicable to the situation found in primary care. For example Jehu (1988) in his book *Beyond Sexual Abuse* reported his experience at the University of Manitoba Sexual Dysfunction Clinic with 51 women found to have a history of sexual abuse. He gives an interview protocol for the assessment of sexual dysfunction which is over 14 pages long. In the preamble to the questionnaire, it is stated that therapists should select and sequence items to suit individual victims, rather than follow it in a rigid or chronological fashion, but it still implies a question-and-answer technique.

Preoccupation with cataloguing and numbering complaints may sometimes be necessary for research purposes, but such an approach is reminiscent of the 'system checklist' that most of us were taught to go through as students, only to observe that experienced clinicians never worked in this fashion. We learnt to abandon the check-list in favour of listening to what was important to the patient – only using questions to make sure that the message as heard was the one told by the patient. Patients tell doctors what is wrong, briefly and succinctly, if they are allowed to do so. Blau (1989) showed that 70 % of patients spoke for less than two minutes when explaining their complaint without interruption to a listening doctor. Clothier (1988) said

> Listen to the complaint of the patient, however tiresome or irrelevant it may seem. He will eventually tell you what is the matter with him . . . It is usually better in terms of both care and time to allow the flow to come to a natural halt from exhaustion of either the speaker or the material.

WHAT IS SEXUAL ABUSE?

A commonly accepted definition of sexual abuse is that given by Kempe and Kempe (1978).

> . . . the involvement of dependent, developmentally-immature children and adolescents in sexual activities they do not comprehend, or that violate the social taboos of family roles.

Children have sexual feelings from a very young age, but sexuality in childhood should be different from that in adult life. When sexual abuse occurs, the roles and boundaries between adult and child have become confused and the trust of the dependent child is betrayed (Furniss, 1983). No child can give 'informed consent' to sexual relationships or activities about which they cannot be knowledgeable. Children may co-operate, agree to the activities, play an active part in the sexual acts and sometimes enjoy them (Yates, 1982) but they cannot give free, informed consent. In any child-adult encounter there is a power imbalance. The misuse of power may include sexual activities in a context of warmth and love, the granting of special status or privileges, bribery, and frequently extreme secrecy, but it continues to be a misuse of the power of the adult over the dependent child. Rape by one adult of another has many parallels with this situation of power imbalance.

The long-term effects of childhood sexual abuse (or of rape) have most frequently been described in patients who are already psychiatrically disturbed. The described effects vary from no ill effects, through to sexual coldness and failure to form lasting emotional relationships, to promiscuity, often associated with alcohol and drug misuse. Those who have been molested have a poor sense of their own worth; they are often depressed and may describe a sense of contamination and dirtiness.

There are few studies of people who have been abused as children but function normally as adults. Tsai *et al.* (1979) compared girls who felt damaged by their experiences (the 'clinical' group) with a matched group who did not. The clinical group tended to have had more frequent molestation of longer duration, with intercourse being more likely. The unaffected group tended to have had more support from family and friends during childhood and had not been blamed for the events; they also tended to have found partners in adult life who were supportive and understanding.

Edwards and Donaldson (1989) used a self-reporting questionnaire to assess the range of commonly reported symptoms experienced by adult survivors of incest. They identified typical stress responses which were identical with those experienced by survivors of other traumatic events. Vulnerability and isolation, fear and anxiety, anger and betrayal, sadness and loss and powerlessness were commonly expressed. Shame, guilt and powerlessness went together with avoidance of activities which aroused recollections of the abuse and a general numbing of responsiveness to the outside world.

PICKING UP THE CLUES

Should patients with problems be asked routinely about prior sexual abuse? Many of the texts and articles written by psychotherapists suggest that they should and state (or imply) that sexual abuse will otherwise be missed. However, when cases are reported in seminars run by the Institute of Psychosexual Medicine, asking questions of this type does not seem productive. There is a danger that, if asked directly, patients may deny such experiences and then find it difficult to retract the denial at a later stage. They may have blocked it out and be unable to recall such events until further work on their problem has made the need for defences less necessary. In addition, care must be taken to ensure that attention is not focused on the abuse such that other, more significant events are ignored. In primary care, patients attend when they choose and they bring to the consultation such matters as they wish to deal with at that particular time. Of course, it is dangerous to collude with a patient who is avoiding looking at part of a problem, but until those events are perceived by the patient as part of the difficulty, no progress can be made. In practice, all that can happen of any benefit is that the therapist must be aware that sexual abuse is common and may be a contributory factor. Doctors must also remember that their own attitudes will influence whether revelations about sexual abuse can take place. They may believe that the account is fantasy material and try to concentrate on the internal world rather than the external reality as perceived by the patient (making statements such as 'all daughters wish to have a sexual relationship with their fathers at some stage of their emotional development'). Some doctors may even indicate to patients that they believe them to have been responsible for the abuse, or they may avoid looking at the material because of the violent emotions that are roused in both the narrator and listener.

In primary care, presentation of sexual abuse is likely to be covert, at least initially. Patients need to try the doctor out to see how their problems will be received. This stratagem may be completely unconscious, or trivial symptoms may be offered to see how the doctor reacts. It is important that the doctor does not become irritated by these apparently time-wasting irrelevances. To do so prevents the patient offering 'While I'm here . . .' and revealing the true nature of the consultation. The patient who attends frequently but never comes to the point of the consultation or makes appointments which are not kept, is having difficulty confronting the doctor openly with a problem that they may feel is shameful.

Primary care physicians are used to looking for non-verbal clues in the consultation. For instance, the patient sitting on the edge of the chair communicates anxiety, and the woman with hair swinging over her face and the loose clothes enveloping her figure is hiding from the world. Similarly there may be particular clues which are suggestive of sexual abuse.

The complaint 'everything always goes wrong for me', or the patient who never manages to make an appointment for her pills which have run out, or the man who sits uncomplainingly in the waiting room overlooked by the receptionist until surgery is finished, are illustrations of the powerlessness of the individual. Similarly, the doctor might question why some patients seem to attract disasters – the woman who marries young to a man who then beats her; she has several children quickly because he threw away her contraceptive pills and pulled out her coil; he goes to prison for assault and she takes in a charming man who cons her out of what money she has and leaves her with a pile of debts in her name – why is she so vulnerable and unable to ask for help in her isolation from the rest of the world? And why does she believe that it is all her fault? She takes the burden of guilt and cannot allow herself to express any anger against those who have treated her badly.

There is also the woman who complains that 'all men are the same' and whose plunging neck-line and tight trousers contradict her cold and remote response to sexual overtures. She is giving a message that outwardly she is a sexualized person but inwardly she avoids responding in a sexual way to prevent the distress of remembering previous experiences. The controlled anger of the woman who married three times in quick succession and obtained substantial financial benefits from each man before setting up on her own with her two over-protected daughters and her scapegoat son, could be interpreted as her continued fury against the father who had ruined her childhood.

Not all these manifestations of distress will be hiding experiences of sexual molestation, but it is much more common than reported. The Children's Society provides a 'safe house' for young runaways. When these runaways were first interviewed, many of them gave vague reasons for leaving home, such as 'I was fed up' or 'I didn't like the way I was treated'. After developing trust in the house staff as many as one in five of these children revealed that they had suffered sexual abuse (The Children's Society, 1989). Given an indication from the doctor that these secrets can be discussed in a non-judgemental way, many more patients will find the courage to divest themselves of their hidden and well-defended problems.

THE MOMENT OF DISCLOSURE

Patients often seek help at moments of crisis and change. A child may disclose abuse because a younger sibling is now thought to be at risk. In one family the three older boys had all been abused by the father for many years. It was only when the youngest, the 'afterthought baby', began receiving threatening overtures from the father that all the older sons got together and decided that they could not tolerate this. They had great difficulty in being heard and believed by the teacher they had chosen for the initial revelation, and by the many authorities with whom they later came in contact. They persevered, however, because of their concern and need to protect their sibling. It would have been understandable if they had retracted since the results were a public furore, the total disruption of the family with imprisonment of the father, the loss of family life by placement with foster parents separately and the loss of friends and relations because of placement away from their city of origin. All of this was only mitigated by their pleasure in retribution and the playing out of their angry feelings towards adults.

A daughter may reveal the abuse when a younger sister is about to supplant her in the special relationship with her father that she has, in part, endured and, in part, enjoyed. Similarly, a developing relationship with a boy outside the enclosed family may be the trigger. Increasing maturity of a long-abused child may evoke a realization that what is happening is not a normal experience for others, or the publicity in the media, the advertizing of contact telephone lines and, more recently, teaching in schools and youth organizations may enable an uncomfortable child to divulge what is going on.

The need to cope with contraception (when no method is ever right!) or with vaginal examination (when the time is never right!) may provide the stimulus for presentation of problems. In a similar way, a new relationship, or the breakdown of an established one can open the door to revelations about experiences which have been buried. The birth of a baby, or the loss by miscarriage or termination, can reawaken the fears of the child within the adult. The masturbatory behaviour of an infant, or the growing sexuality of the adolescent, can be presented to the doctor as an inappropriately enormous and worrying problem requiring the unravelling of the underlying secrets. One man presented his recollections of molestation by his father from whom he had been estranged for many years. It is interesting that he was not able to recall and talk about his experiences until the death of his father. Then he was able to reveal his irrational fears that the mantle of exploitation would be passed on to him on his father's death, although up to that time he had led an entirely conventional life.

Recently, the publicity on television and in the papers has reawakened the memories of many patients who thought that they had dealt with that part of their past by burying it deep. They may suddenly present with this history in order to make sense of it in their now-adult selves. Some may use it as a defence to avoid looking for other reasons why they may be having difficulties with relationships. Others may not be affected, but be unable to understand why they should not be feeling outrage and anger against the perpetrator – after all this is what they are supposed to be feeling according to the media! A few patients will be so damaged by their experiences that little help is possible.

THE RESPONSIBILITY OF THE PRIMARY CARE DOCTOR

Why look at these difficult and threatening problems within primary care? Surely there are people who are specially trained to cope with this type of problem?

The first impulse of the doctor faced with these revelations will be 'Where can I send this patient?'. The patients, however, often do not want to go anywhere else; they want to be met with a calm acceptance that it is possible to learn to cope with such problems and, perhaps more importantly, be shown that they are not so despoiled that their doctor cannot touch them. It takes enough courage to tell one person, and that person they may have needed to 'try out' first. The thought of telling someone else, a stranger, these awful things, or worse still, being referred to a specialist as though they were ill or mad is often out of the question. So primary care is faced with such problems and we have to learn how to do our best to deal with them.

REFERENCES

Blau, J. N. (1989) Time to Let the Patient Speak. *Br. Med. J.*, **298**, 39.

The Children's Society (1989) *Young Runaways: Findings from Britain's First Safe House*, The Children's Society, Edward Rudolph House, London.

Clothier, C. (1988) *The Patient's Dilemma*, Nuffield Provincial Hospitals Trust, London.

Edwards, P. W. and Donaldson, M. A. (1989) Assessment of Symptoms in Adult Survivors of Incest. *Child Abuse & Neglect*, **13**, 101–10.

Furniss, T. (1983) Mutual Influence and Interlocking Professional – Family Process in the Treatment of Child Sexual Abuse and Incest. *Child Abuse & Neglect*, **7**, 207–23.

Jehu, D. (1988) *Beyond Sexual Abuse*, John Wiley & Sons Ltd, Chichester.

Kempe, R. S. and Kempe, C. H. (1978) *Child Abuse*, Fontana/Open Books, London.

Tsai, M., Feldman-Summers, S. and Edgar, M. (1979) Childhood Molestation: Variables Related to Differential Impacts on Psychosocial Functioning in Adult Women. *Journal of Abnormal Psychology*, **88**, 407–17.

Yates, A. (1982) Children Eroticized by Incest. *American Journal of Psychiatry*, **139** (4), 482–5.

2

What is normal?

The publicity of the last few years has permitted discussion of sexual abuse, a previously taboo subject. Patients now expect their doctors to know about the normal as well as the abnormal. They bring their fears and questions to those they view as having expert knowledge.

Mr J had finished talking to the doctor about his indigestion. While the doctor waited, expecting him to get up and go, he looked at his trouser leg and picked off imaginary pieces of fluff. He took a deep breath, looked past the doctor's ear and said 'Do you think I should stop giving my little girl her bath before she goes to bed?' The doctor looked puzzled and enquiring, not having any idea what this was about. Mr J went on to explain that he and his wife had been talking about how awful all this business was – about sexual abuse. He had said how he could not understand how anyone could hurt a child. His wife had remarked that it might be him being accused of doing things he should not, after all, he was always cuddling Dawn and he gave her baths and dressed her for bed. He looked very worried and concerned.

The doctor is in a dilemma; in such a situation a number of interpretations are possible. Should the patient's fears be taken at face value? Is it just that with the increase in publicity about childhood sexual abuse, parents are now genuinely afraid to show their natural love and tenderness for their children in case it is misinterpreted? Or is this man expressing his own worry about his feelings, fearful that they may become uncontrollable? Or is his wife worried that he will not be able to control his tenderness – or could she be jealous of the depth of emotion he exhibits and feels excluded from the relationship between father and daughter?

PERSONAL EXPERIENCE IS NOT ENOUGH

The doctor has feelings about this situation as well. Given that doctors have received little or no professional training about what is normal behaviour between parents and children, the response will depend very much on personal experience. A doctor, brought up in a home where nudity is accepted as normal, where bathroom and bedroom doors are not locked and physical contact between members of the family is frequent and acceptable will have one set of standards. Another, raised in a home where everyone is seen fully attired in clothes or an enveloping dressing gown, where the bathroom door is not only locked but nobody approaches it if it is thought to be occupied, bedrooms are private territory and bodily contact is limited and formalized – this doctor will have a very different set of standards. These parameters of 'normal behaviour' can be modified by encounters with other family systems when visiting friends and relatives, and by later experiences which cause a re-evaluation of the internalized family standard. Very often, however, these standards have never been examined or evaluated, and the doctor responds with only personal knowledge as a guide. Statements such as 'Goodness me, you mustn't worry about that, I bathed my children until they were too old to need it any more' or 'I think your daughter is getting a little old for that sort of thing – better to leave it to her mother' are particularly unhelpful. If the internal standards of the patient and the doctor do not coincide, the patient will feel confused by the advice. He will usually ignore it as irrelevant, but could try to comply which would make him feel uncomfortable.

So how can the doctor determine what is a 'normal relationship' between parent and child? A search through the literature available in a medical library will give an enormous amount of information about what is abnormal. Normality is always more difficult to define. Information about how the child goes through various stages of emotional development is available in standard textbooks and from this deductions can be made about the interactions between parent and child.

THE DEVELOPMENT OF SENSUALITY

Family bonds of love and caring develop from the passionate feelings between the young child and the parent. Most children are encouraged to give expression to their intense feelings of love and it is natural that when they first wish for a physical expression of that love that this should be directed at the parent. For children to develop into healthy, loving and sensual adults, incestuous fantasies are necessary, but the expression of these yearnings needs to be controlled by the parents. Clear, unambiguous, signals from parents as to what is acceptable are necessary for healthy emotional development. Within the family are three elements of sensuality: the parents' own sex life; the child's developing sensual feelings; and the tendency by the parents to re-experience their own childhood sensuality in the relationship with the child.

The way in which the child's sensual feelings are kept in control by the parent is absorbed and retained by the child. As the child approaches the watershed of adolescence, biological changes increase sensual feelings towards the parent of the opposite sex. The continuing controls of the parent are very necessary here, balancing admiration of the developing sexual person against the adolescent need for privacy in order to become an individual separate from the family. Parental tasks are made easier when clear early response patterns have been retained by the child. When the teenagers turn into parents themselves, these internal controls are used again as the parent expresses physical love for a child, without exposing them to sexual seduction.

It follows from this that anything that goes wrong with the constraints leads to a situation fraught with danger. Where there is a lack of sexual fulfilment in the marital relationship and the child is seen as a substitute for marital loving, a physical expression of love from the child will be encouraged disproportionately and may lead to sexual physical interactions. This is most likely when the parent suffered in early childhood from a lack of love or care, or the loss of a parent, or had no opportunity to learn an internal regulation of incestuous feelings. There may be an inability to comprehend the need for control, or to withstand the desire, and love is expressed in a sexual way.

Consider again the situation presented by Mr J and his query – what exactly is his problem?

> The doctor acknowledged Mr J's feelings by saying that most fathers enjoyed bathing their daughters; how did he feel about it? He said that they enjoyed messing about with the water and the flannel – sometimes Dawn got a bit too giggly and silly and then he had to bring her down to earth again.

Mr J's attitude indicated to the doctor that there need be no concern about lack of control and that Mr J did not appear to be exploiting the child's love in order to substitute for any lack in his own sexual life either now or in the past.

> And what about his wife? Mr J said that she had had Dawn all day and wanted a bit of a break. She had always been pleased that he wanted to take over in the evening and put Dawn to bed. He had been quite surprised that she had even thought in that way.
>
> Did he think she might be a bit jealous? He was getting the 'fun' time and she was shut out from the closeness? Mr J thought about that and acknowledged that his wife always seemed 'a bit huffy and distant' when he came down after putting Dawn to bed. 'Perhaps she feels a bit neglected, although I always want to give her a cuddle when I come down and she always tells me to give over.'
>
> The doctor said that perhaps his wife needed the cuddle before he gave his time to Dawn? Mr J was indignant – 'she knows she always comes first with me!'. The doctor looked at him and felt his anger at the criticism subside as he recognized the possibility. The doctor closed the consultation with 'Why not talk some more with your wife about it all and sort out what feels right for you both?'.

Mr J had become alarmed by the force of feeling expressed by his wife. He felt he had done something wrong but had not discovered what this was. The mention of incest feelings or fantasies provoke panic, guilt and denial. The feelings parents have towards their child reawaken the memories from early childhood of closeness, of rejection, of intense desire towards the parent and realization that they alter the previous duality of marital relationships. Without discovering exactly what Mr J was concerned about, a lecture on 'normal relationships' (even if the doctor knew what they were) would have been useless.

SIBLING RELATIONSHIPS

Incestuous fantasies and feelings may be given more overt expression in relationships between siblings. Little has been written about this but a useful account of how to differentiate between exploitation and normal sexual exploration is given in de Jong (1989). The child's curiosity about bodies can lead to exciting sexualized play. This may be more tolerated than a similar relationship between parent and child, unless there are big age differences, and the younger child is exploited for the purposes of the older one. Yet if the erotic feelings are not controlled, later adult relationships may be jeopardized. Sometimes when a girl marries her brother's best friend, or a young man his sister's friend, or someone who closely resembles a sibling, problems ensue.

Mrs S was a naval wife. Her husband had recently returned from a tour away for several months and she could not bear him to touch her. It would have been easy to attribute her problems to resentment over the separation (they had not been married long before he was posted) but careful listening revealed another problem.

When her husband had returned she was overjoyed to see him again but found she had a strange uncomfortable feeling when sitting looking at him at home – as though he was the wrong man who had come home. At first she put this down to their separation and that they had not known each other for long before he had gone away – she thought they needed to get to know each other again. The feeling of strangeness had persisted and she was beginning to think that she must be unhinged – she felt he was not the same man who had gone away.

She was asked to go through what was different about him, and during this catalogue of mainly negative observations, remarked that he had grown a moustache. She stopped and the doctor waited. A long silence. Mrs S burst out 'He looks just like

> D now he's grown a moustache!'. She was able to go on to explain that D was her brother, four years older. And with more difficulty she began to release her intense sexual feelings about him. She related how close they had been, how distraught she was when he left home and how angry she had been with him when he returned home for a visit, with a new moustache, and a new life from which she was excluded.

Mrs S had unconsciously chosen a husband who resembled her dearly-loved brother. When he too left (rejected her) and returned with the symbolic moustache of a separate life, her previous anger was re-awakened and the confusion between her feelings for her brother and her feelings for her husband prevented a normal sexual relationship. She had not been aware of the normality of sensual feelings in childhood and adolescence and had suppressed her early emotions because of guilty feelings that they were abnormal. If Mrs S had had a better awareness of normality, she might have been able to recognize the resemblance between her brother and her husband, and her feelings for both, at an earlier stage.

SOCIAL ATTITUDES AND PARENTING

Originally, images of sexual abuse in families were those of a relationship between father and adolescent daughter which was basically loving and had taken an inappropriate sexual form. Sexual abuse of young children or even infants is a much less comfortable image. It is understandable if parents panic and refuse to recognize this. As a society we are still in the early stages of coping with child abuse. Kempe and Kempe (1978) described various stages of the way in which abuse is viewed. The first three stages occur early during recognition of the problem. Denial that it could happen at all is followed by a recognition of only the more florid manifestations. Then, as severe cases are recognized, more subtle forms of abuse can be acknowledged.

These three phases of viewing sexual abuse have already been traversed in the recognition of physical abuse. At first there was a denial that injuries could ever have been caused by the parents. Second, a recognition of the bruised and battered child with multiple fractures as a victim of parental violence became accepted. Third, more minor physical ill-treatment then become indentifiable. Sexual abuse is hovering between the stages of denial and recognition of only the most obvious cases. Much of the sexual abuse of infants and young children is anal rather than vaginal, and it is becoming apparent that it is possibly as common in boys as in girls (Hobbs and Wynne, 1986; 1987).

It is tempting to try to distance ourselves from such abuse by assuming that the people who do such things are unlike ourselves. As we have had to do with physical abuse, this behaviour must be understood in the context of the interactions between parents and children.

The publicity about extreme forms of child sexual abuse has made many parents anxious and guilty about their previously hidden emotions. Because of this some people have difficulty in accepting the beneficial effects of demonstrations of affection between members of a family. In infancy and childhood, close bonds and physical expression of love are essential to normal emotional maturation. As the child matures, gradual freedom from these bonds must be achieved. Incestuous longings must not be allowed to take over and risk harming the child, but need to be recognized and controlled. Loving relationships between family members can then be enjoyed, even with the erotic elements, without panic and guilt.

REFERENCES

Hobbs, C. J. and Wynne, J. M. (1986) Buggery in Childhood, a Common Syndrome of Child Abuse. *Lancet*, **ii**, 792–6.

Hobbs, C. J. and Wynne, J. M. (1987) Management of Sexual Abuse. *Archives Diseases in Childhood*, **62** (ii), 182–7.

de Jong, A. R. (1989) Sexual Interactions among Siblings and Cousins: Experimentation or Exploitation? *Child Abuse & Neglect*, **13**, 271–9.

Kempe, R. S. and Kempe, C. H. (1978) *Child Abuse*, Fontana/Open Books, London.

3

Adolescent confusions

The erotic nature of the emotions between young children and their parents may be hidden away, and discussion of such emotions is a taboo area. At adolescence the emerging sexuality is a common cause of problems and, at the same time, easier to recognize because of its overt nature. Early adolescence with its physical changes and re-awakened erotic emotions is a critical phase of development at a time when conflicts between parents and children are common. The ardour of the child will disinter unresolved sexual anxieties in the parents, which in turn affect the ability of the child to cope with the emotional load.

Mrs B rang her doctor in great distress; something awful had happened, she must talk to the doctor today about it. When she arrived, the normally well-turned out woman looked distraught and unkempt. She shook and wept with anger as she recounted her story.

She had returned from a business trip earlier than expected and had surprised her daughter and her husband in bed together. She had remarried two years ago, to a man 20 years her junior. She had gone off on a business trip, as she often did, leaving her 15-year-old daughter and the step-father to 'look after each other'(!)

Now that she knew what was going on, she couldn't understand how she had ignored the sexual innuendoes between the two of them – the daughter's provocative behaviour with her husband, and the competition between her daughter and herself to always be the best-dressed and the most attractive. Her daughter had stolen her make-up, her clothes and now her husband.

Nowhere in the account was any blame attached to the man. He was hardly mentioned. All the story was about the conflict between daughter and mother. The mother in her heightened state of sexuality in a new relationship had been unable to openly acknowledge her daughter's growing need to be a sexual individual. The daughter, from being the close companion and emotional support of her mother in the aftermath of a messy divorce, had been cast aside for a new, highly-charged relationship. The denial of the daughter's emotional needs and her emerging sexual feelings had led her to compete in a more and more provocative way in order to obtain the emotional succour she had lost when her mother remarried, and to demonstrate that she too was a sexually-attractive woman. (It is perhaps symptomatic of cultural values that the sexual approach from a minor to a man, who is married to her mother and is ten years older than herself, was not rejected and controlled as it should have been.)

PHYSICAL AND EMOTIONAL CHANGES

Parents often express their bewilderment at what is happening in adolescence. The alarming biological changes that occur are frequently accompanied by moodiness and sudden changes from 'almost adult' behaviour to marked childishness. The early adolescent has to find the way through all these feelings and experiences and often finds it a confusing and frightening task.

The boy may want to hide the evidence of wet dreams, not just because of the difficulty of coming to terms with his lack of control over a new physical happening, but also because the dreams may involve women he recognizes as symbolizing his mother or sister. The development of breasts and the onset of menstruation provide girls with similar dilemmas. They can enter the adult 'women's world' but are fearful of what this entails. They want to keep their childish relationship with their father and keep these changes secret, while at the same time wanting the father to know that they are now sexual women.

At times like these, parents are always in the wrong – if they comment on the physical changes of adolescence they are accused of causing embarrassment, if they do not, they are accused of not caring.

PARENTS AND OUTSIDE RELATIONSHIPS

The importance of relationships developing outside the family causes even more secretive behaviour. Parents who have an unsatisfactory sexual life of their own tend to react to their children's exploration of the outside world of relationships in two ways. They either become very restrictive to shore up their own defences, or become too encouraging and permissive in order to gain a vicarious satisfaction from their offsprings' sexuality. Both of these make it very difficult for adolescents to come to their own decisions about their sexual and emotional development.

H, a very attractive, immaculately-dressed blonde girl, attended the doctor with overbreathing attacks. It had been quite difficult to discover why these attacks should be occurring. H came from a well-off home, was attending college with the blessing of her parents and no trace of any difficulty could be found. It was all too nice. Mother attended with H to express her concern and the doctor was struck by the resemblance between mother and daughter – they looked more like sisters.

In a later consultation with H alone, the doctor commented on this to H and was taken aback at the sudden release of emotion, like a pressure cooker letting off steam. H described how she hated her mother, who was always so reasonable. If H wanted to do anything that did not fit in with the family plans, her mother would explain to her how H surely would not want to upset the family arrangements, and manoeuvre her into agreeing. Her father took all the decisions about what they were going to do and treated H as a sort of extension of her mother who would always want to do the same.

She said she felt suffocated by the family, and wept with anger as she explained how she felt she was betraying them; they gave her everything. If she had a friend, especially if male, they would invite him to their house and overwhelm him with kindness.

This patient was not allowed to show any unpleasant emotions: nothing to disturb the equanimity of the household. Adolescent rebellion, passion or anger were not permitted and H had been corralled into the obedient resemblance of her controlled mother. Her emerging sexual feelings were damped down by the parents taking over any of her male relationships and sanitizing them. It was understandable that she felt suffocated and suffered from overbreathing attacks.

In subsequent consultations the patient was able to talk more openly about her father.

H described how he controlled all aspects of life for her and her mother. He had to be consulted about what clothes they wore, what they did, who they saw. He treated them with courtly grace but his word was law. H had always accepted that this was how fathers were until she had gone to college and discovered alternative patterns of parenting. Now she wanted to take her own decisions and to be a 'woman' not a child. She had always tried to please him but had never managed to obtain any expression of approval. He never hugged her like she had seen some fathers do, he just got her to stand before him for inspection – and always found something to criticize.

This girl had no acknowledgement of her growing maturity and sexuality. Her father kept any frightening sexuality well-hidden and treated both daughter and wife as possessions to be polished and presented to the world. The doctor could only speculate privately about the sexual difficulties of H's parents.

THE DOCTOR AND THE ADOLESCENT

Other consultations may be more difficult and confronting for the doctor. Adolescents are always challenging and often put doctors in a quandary as to the role expected of them. Because the adolescent swings from being a child to an (almost) adult, the doctor has to modify the response accordingly from parental reaction to equal adult, from acceptance to guardianship.

C, a 14-year-old with a pale face and dressed in clothes that made her look younger was brought to her GP by her mother who looked tight-lipped and angry.

The story was that C had missed her last three periods; her mother had taken a sample of urine to the chemist and a positive pregnancy test had been obtained. The dates would have made her 14-weeks pregnant. C looked as if it was nothing to do with her. The doctor obtained permission from her to do an examination – which was performed with C lying there, legs apart, completely detached from the proceedings. (The doctor noted the reaction but did not think that the time was right for any interpretation.) The uterus was not enlarged and the doctor was puzzled.

Practical arrangements were made with C and her mother for an ultrasound scan. Now that the anxiety and urgency felt by both doctor and mother about a possible advanced pregnancy had been relieved, the doctor felt able to ask the mother to leave the room. When alone with C little was achieved except to obtain the information that C did have a boyfriend, but that she had not done anything 'like that' with him, he was only a daft lad, into drinking with his mates and talking big. If she was pregnant, she was keeping the baby, her mum didn't care about her anyway. She could not be diverted from a catalogue of complaints about her mother and her step-father.

When she returned (with a negative pregnancy test and an empty uterus on the scan), the relationship between C and the doctor was easier. C was encouraged to talk about why she had thought she might be pregnant. She had told her mother as soon as she had missed her first period, but her mother had taken no notice. She had then taken to staying out later than was allowed by her strict step-father and causing all sorts of rows at home. The detailed description of the rows kept the doctor at a distance for some time, and the consultation was eventually terminated with the arrangement of another one to follow.

C cancelled her next appointment, and the one after that, but did turn up once the doctor had phoned her personally to fix another appointment (after a long session with the mother who was finding C very difficult to cope with). C looked less assured and defiant. Her mother had suggested that C should go and stay with her grandmother for a bit, as they were all getting on so badly at home. Hesitantly the story emerged: she liked staying with her Gran; she let her do what she liked and Gran went out a lot in the evenings. But her own Dad was home now, living with Gran (he worked abroad for several months at a time) and would want her 'to do things' with him. After a long silence C told of the gradual progression from affectionate play to more intimate fondling and, finally, to full penetration. She had 'let' him do it because she wanted his love and attention.

The doctor discussed with C what to do next. C was keen for Social Services to be involved. With her permission her mother was telephoned and asked to come and see the doctor. The mother had suspected something of the sort (and was ready to believe anything of her ex-husband towards whom she still felt very bitter). She was happy to have Social Services involved and obviously relieved to share the responsibility of doing something about her daughter.

The doctor had been alerted to a problem by the original examination (C had shut the doctor out from her emotions about the vaginal examination) and again when C was asked why she thought she might be pregnant. Failing to turn up for appointments is a common indicator that the patient is suffering from feelings of a lack of power and is in need of defences, as is the uncommunicative behaviour so prevalent in adolescence. The acceptance of C's behaviour and continuing expressions of care from the doctor enabled C to tell her story. Apparent uncritical acceptance and lack of embarrassment are important aids to prising a history from a reluctant, anti-authoritarian adolescent. The door needs to be open to receive the emotions which are confusing and often paralysing for the victim. The commonest of these emotions is guilt.

Why did C feel so guilty? The desire of an adolescent for the parent of the opposite sex is well-documented and easily accepted. What is more difficult to accept is the sexual excitement and enjoyment. Anyone stimulated sexually can either shut off all sensations and not react at all, or be aroused. The forbidden nature of the encounter only serves to heighten the excitement. But, because of this excitement, guilt that the situation must in some way be the fault of the victim, becomes accepted. 'She led him on' or 'she was asking for it' are frequent public statements heard. However, the adult is in a position of power over the child, and with that power should come responsibility.

THE ABSENT MOTHER

The other predominant emotion expressed is anger at the mother, and this anger is not just towards a sexual rival for the attentions of the male adult. Frequently the abused child will not mention the mother, or complain that she was absent or uncaring. It is as though the role of the mother is to help to control and direct the emerging sexuality of the adolescent into an acceptable role, and to provide the correct focus for the male sexuality. The fantasy is that the male is constantly rampant and only the mother can provide the controls, but the reality is that the acceptable expressions of controlled sensual contact with children – breast-feeding, kissing, cuddling and bathing – seem to be inappropriately interpreted by the parents in families where sexual molestation occurs.

Mothers undoubtedly play a significant role in the emotional life of the developing child and adolescent. The emphasis on the popular image of sexual abuse being between a loving father and his teenage daughter ignores the significance of the absence of the mother figure. If the mother intrudes into this imagined picture, the fantasy fades under the harsh spotlight of sordid reality, the reality of exploitation and violation.

ONE PATIENT OR TWO?

Adolescents usually attend either with their mothers or the mother comes to complain about, or on behalf of, the daughter. The cases described earlier illustrate some of the difficulties inherent in seeing more than one patient at a time. There is a temptation to treat one as 'the patient' and to collude with the other. It is essential that both are made to feel that the doctor will listen to each in a serious doctoring way.

At some stage in the consultation it should be possible to see each of them separately. Usually this can be done early in the consultation with a promise to talk subsequently with the excluded one (preferably the parent as the adolescent is nominally the patient, at least initially).

It is essential that no information is divulged to any third party without permission except when urgent protection is required (when they may have to be told that this is necessary). Assurances about confidentiality are often sought and should always be given with this proviso. Comments which might be painful to the other participant can then be divulged to the doctor in confidence.

In a one-to-one consultation, it is easier to note the interactions between doctor and patient and make use of them. Where two patients are present, much of the doctor's attention is taken up with observing the interaction between the patients and it is more difficult to use this interplay in an interpretative and uncritical way. When two patients are present, one may answer for the other, or be unable to tolerate a silence.

Difficulties are also produced by any disliked characteristics such as selfishness or intolerance possessed by one family member and unconsciously projected onto another member of the family who can then be overtly disliked or criticized for those characteristics. It is rarely possible to point out this projection in a joint consultation. Seeing each separately allows consideration of the individual problems which each is experiencing.

The adolescent must be made to feel that the doctor is not just another parental figure, whilst the parent must be able to accept that the doctor understands the dilemmas and difficulties of parenthood.

4

Abuse as a 'visiting card'

The publicity about sexual abuse in childhood has allowed a number of patients to come forward with their stories of sexual abuse. The doctor knows that a history of sexual abuse can have serious consequences for the individual, and will often be tempted to concentrate on the abuse and not to look at other harmful episodes and feelings. The words 'sexual abuse' become a password for taking action, any action, in any direction. That this action may not be particularly appropriate is lost in the panic of 'having to do something'.

It is easy for a patient who uses the complaint of sexual abuse as a 'visiting card' to become labelled and categorized. Other emotional problems which are of more importance to that patient are then not examined. Doctors and other professionals find it very difficult to overcome their natural inclinations to examine the sexual abuse episode in depth. We are told from all directions that sexual abuse is a deeply disturbing experience and causes scars which last for life. However, without diminishing the importance of such events, unless the abuse episode is perceived as important by the patient it is a cul-de-sac down which we venture only to be frustrated to find there is no progress.

THE MOTHER WHO DID NOT CARE

Often cases present when the need of the patient to be a mother reawakens feelings about the patient's own deficient mothering.

E arrived early and anxious after referral from the Health Visitor, who thought she had 'post-natal depression' and had mentioned 'sexual abuse'. She was a tiny, dark-haired woman with a tired grey face almost concealed by the up-turned collar of a huge grey raincoat. She sat hunched in the chair and her misery was suffocating. She said that her pregnancy had been a nightmare and no-one had known why. If the child had been a girl she would have killed herself; she could not have let a girl have her bad experiences. She gave the doctor a long and prepared story.

Briefly, after the suicide of her father, her mother could not cope with her and a younger brother. She had been sent to stay with an aunt. Because she was homesick and wept at night, she was allowed to sleep with the aunt and her husband. He had been kind and gentle and she had enjoyed his fondling in bed, until one night when he had tried to put his finger inside her and she had cried out with pain. There had been a tremendous row and the aunt had packed her cases in the morning and taken E. home. When her mother heard what had happened there was another storm 'everyone shouting but no-one spoke to me, I did not know what I had done, but no-one talked to me for weeks and my mother did not care that I had been hurt.'

The doctor clumsily pursued the sexual experience but was dismissed with impatience. Didn't the doctor hear what she was saying? Her mother had not cared. She had just not bothered.

The release of these angry feelings during the next few

sessions with a doctor trained in psychosexual medicine enabled the patient to come to terms with them. As a result, she was then able to move forward in the development of her own maternal feelings towards her own child.

In many areas there are groups set up to support and help people to come to terms with what has happened to them. Individual help is less widely available, although some psychologists and psychiatrists have set up rehabilitation programmes for victims arising from their own interests in the problem. There is often pressure on the doctor to refer any patient to locally available facilities, specifically to look at the prior sexual abuse.

To enter patients like E into a rehabilitation programme or to make any other routine response to sexual abuse disclosure, is at best a waste of time, at worst a reinforcement of their difficulties. The anger towards mothers who the patients feel did not care enough to prevent these (awful) things happening, can be so enormous that it blots out all other feelings and shouts to be heard.

CONTESTING FOR MOTHER'S ATTENTION

U's mother originally attended with her husband, complaining of agoraphobic symptoms preventing her from going to work. The family had been patients with the practice for many years and were well regarded as sensible but a bit over-concerned about the health of their children. It was only on the mother's fifth attendance that the real problem at home emerged: she could not go out because of what U might do or say. U had leant out of the bedroom window last night and shouted at the top of her voice that her step-father was having sex with her.

Arrangements were made to see U (their 14-year-old-daughter). Her mother was emphatic that she would rather the doctor saw her on her own, and when U arrived she said that she did not want her mother there. The doctor sat silently, just nodding or 'um-ming' as U launched into a diatribe about how awful her parents were. Her mother had married that man; he was horrible, he walked around with no clothes on in their house; he tried to kiss her and do things. The doctor was trying hard not to become too alarmed by all this, and not too overwhelmed by the girl's anger. With a little prompting of 'can you tell me a bit more about that?' and 'how did that make you feel?' a more complete story emerged.

The mother had U as a single parent and had met and married this man nine years ago. There was a daughter of eight who U thought was always favoured above herself. Her step-father was always cuddling and kissing her sister; it was disgusting. When he tried to do it to her she screamed and shouted; she was not going to allow him to treat her like that. When she was asked what she would like to happen, she said her step-father should leave with her sister, leaving herself and her mother together. Once on the subject of her mother, it was difficult to stop. It became clear that she wanted the exclusive attention of her mother.

It would have been very easy to have jumped in and assumed that this girl was at risk of sexual abuse. It took time and patience to unravel the story sufficiently to be fairly sure that this was not the case and that the difficulty lay with her anger for her mother whom she saw as abandoning her in favour of her step-father and step-sister. She had discovered that her accusations against her step-father greatly alarmed her mother and had made her mother stay at home with her over the school summer holiday. The punishment she had received for her bad behaviour had reinforced her anger and sense of injustice. It eventually emerged that the behaviour had been triggered by overhearing her mother talking about having another baby – another contestant for her mother's attention was more than she could bear. After discussion with U and the parents, this family were referred to the community psychiatric nurse who was able to visit them regularly at home and work with them individually over many months.

POWERLESS TO CHOOSE

Listening to find out what the problem is for that particular patient and not allowing distraction by the awfulness of sexual abuse, is the most important skill that can be offered to the patient.

> Mr and Mrs Y attended together. He did all the talking. She must have some therapy to get rid of her hang-ups. (Despite his Greek name and appearance his colloquial English was excellent). When they had first married three years ago everything was fine, but over the last two months she would not let him touch her; it was all the fault of that evil man, her step-father, who had interfered with her. The doctor wondered why the problem had only just started but was brushed aside by the husband; the problem was urgent, it was time for them to start a family.
>
> With some difficulty the doctor managed to arrange to see the wife alone for another consultation. Mrs Y, a slim, attractive English girl told a different story. She had met her husband while working as an accountant on their hotel business. They had married, and while he was learning the business everything had been marvellous. Now he, and his extended family, expected her to give up her career, help in the hotel and raise lots of children. She could not begin to talk about it; they

could not comprehend that she wanted a career of her own, they would not listen. It had brought back memories of her step-father. Her mother had remarried after a stormy divorce, when she was eleven. Her step-father was domineering and had always insisted that she should kiss him and used to put his hands over her body in a way she disliked. She has been trying to tell her husband how she felt powerless and threatened in the same way but he did not understand what she meant. At the end of this consultation Mrs Y said that she did not want to attend again, she must work it out for herself.

She was seen several months later for an unrelated condition and said that she had left her husband. There had been a big row when she finally made him understand. He had said she was of no use to him if she would not help in the hotel or have children; he would get another wife who would, and she had left him. She said she was older and wiser and could see how she had been swept off her feet. She could acknowledge her inner needs to be looked after as well as her desires to be independent and said that she would be more cautious next time.

Mrs Y had experiences as a teenager which had made her feel threatened and powerless to say to her step-father that she did not want him to touch her like that. Her memories of lack of power had been re-awakened when she felt unable to withstand the pressure from her husband and his family to follow a life style which she found unacceptable. Her only weapon to prevent this happening was to withdraw from intercourse. She had, perhaps unconsciously, allowed her husband to misinterpret the episodes in her teens as a reason for her withdrawal; she was unable to state her real reasons clearly enough for him to understand. For two months this had proved a potent defence against her husband's advances.

Only when she discussed this with a trained doctor could she acknowledge what she was doing and gain the confidence to express her wishes clearly and without equivocation. She came to her own conclusions that she was not prepared to change her desired way of life for this man, nor to continue the subterfuge of hiding behind what had been labelled as previous sexual abuse. She was usually a self-assured young woman confident in her own ability to run her own life. She only needed a short consultation to give her considerable insight into the situation and to decide not to be dependent but to sort it out for herself.

LISTENING FOR THE REAL PROBLEM

Other patients may prove far more difficult and demanding for the doctor.

> V looked much younger than her 23 years. Recently registered, she sat carefully in the spare chair in the consulting room, as far away from the doctor as possible. 'I'm so glad you're a woman doctor' she said, 'I can't talk to men at all, I'm really terrified of them.' She gave a rehearsed history of drug abuse and her rehabilitation programme. There was a silence. The doctor asked 'What can I do for you?'. Another silence. Then she launched into a long story about her financial difficulties. The doctor could not see what all this had to do with her and becoming impatient, said so. 'But I have to go and see this man about this money business, and I can't.' V wailed. She revealed that she thought he might make sexual advances to her and she could not cope with that.
>
> Eventually after much hesitation, V told of her experiences with a therapist when she was a teenage drug addict. Her parents had arranged the therapy and after a while the (male) therapist had

instigated sexual intercourse at the end of every session with him. At this point she looked directly at the doctor for the first time. 'You are just like all the others, you don't believe it happened! But it did, it did.'

The doctor felt very uncomfortable, for the thought that this might be a transference fantasy had just gone through her mind. She felt that her relationship with V, so tenuous, needed kid gloves, but she could not avoid this confrontation. As honestly as possible, she explained exactly why she might have doubts and said 'But it really doesn't matter whether it happened or not, what matters is how it has made you feel that men only regard you as an available sexual object with no power to choose for yourself'. V ignored the explanation of doubts and seized on the powerless image. This was the real problem; this is why she had been unable to resist drug taking, why she could not sort out her financial problems, why she thought men only wanted her for one thing.

Of course, this patient's problem was not as simple as that. However, if the doctor had had to protest that she did believe her; that she had been betrayed by her trust and relationship with a therapist into sexual intercourse and the discussion had focused on how terrible that was, the real problem for that patient at that time would have been missed. It was, in fact, possible at a later date to go back to this episode and sort out how she felt about it, but that was not the difficulty with which she had attended on this occasion. Her feelings were those of being a powerless pawn in some bigger game. She thought she would be punished for any attempt to stand up for herself by being forced to submit to the desires of 'man'. She had come to see a 'powerful woman' for help in the confrontation.

THE TEMPTATIONS OF ROUTINE

The feeling of panic and of being overwhelmed that a doctor often experiences when sexual abuse is presented can inhibit proper thought. It is tempting to escape into a routine: all patients with a history of abuse must have in-depth therapy – mustn't they? And, of course, it must be done by an 'expert' – mustn't it? It can't be my job to sort this out!

However, the time to help a patient with a problem is when it is presented. A patient may never summon up the courage to tell anyone else, especially if the doctor demonstrates that the problem is so dreadful by passing it on to an outsider. In addition, as shown in the previous cases discussed, the problem for the patient may not actually be the abuse. It may be the parenting, or the self-image; or difficulties in the present relationship where it is easier to blame an earlier experience than to deal with the present emotions inhibiting sexual response.

The seductive nature of the complaint of sexual abuse, with its undertones of horror and excitement, can have a powerful effect on the doctor. Recognition of the intense personal reaction in the physician enables him or her to avoid being led up the garden path by the sensational aspects of the story. Staying with the patient's emotional distress enables the messages, hidden behind the visiting card of sexual abuse, to emerge and illuminate the true source of the problem for that patient at that time.

5

Denial, guilt and excitement

One of the most difficult areas to cope with and stay with is the emotional distress produced by the ideas of sexual abuse. The most frequent reaction of family members and professionals is denial. A common theme runs through accounts given by people who have been ill-used in this way. Repeatedly we hear that they told of their experiences and were not heard, or they were accused of lying or fantasizing. One woman said that when she tried to tell her previous doctor about what had happened to her as a child, he had patted her on the hand and said it was normal for children to have fantasies about marrying their parents – not what she had told him at all!

Patients themselves may deny what has happened both consciously and unconsciously. The knowledge can be hidden behind defences that are necessary to protect patients from their feelings of guilt and shame. But how can there be guilt unless the victim feels in some way responsible for what has happened?

There seems to be two main sides to the acceptance of responsibility by the victim: sharing a secret relationship with the abuser and trying to cope with sexual arousal.

THE SECRET RELATIONSHIP

The first is the secret sharing of a special relationship. The perpetrator frequently emphasizes to the child that no-one should know, that they have a special secret, and that this cannot be revealed without the child being blamed. The behaviour of the adult during the sexual episodes, when there may be tenderness or expression of concern, contrasted with the uncaring, often over-strict and punitive behaviour exhibited in public, further serves to confuse the child into being unable to reveal what is happening.

Often, when adults are talking about their childhood experiences, they express their bewilderment and their impression of unreality about what was happening in private when the public reality was so different. This dream-like quality to the events has increased the difficulties of differentiation between fantasy and actual events. Accurate description of sexual acts by children who could not otherwise know such details (such as the taste of ejaculate) can effectively discriminate between fact and fantasy. Reports from adults remembering past events are necessarily less accurate and may be modified by later experiences. But in adults the need for rigorous standards of truth are much less and the belief of the patient that violation has occurred is sufficient for the work to proceed.

The activities of the abusing adults fulfill only their need for sexual satisfaction and such actions ignore the child's need to grow and develop at its own pace. The power is with the adult and the child loses its sense of self-esteem. As the child's sense of worthlessness is increased the acceptance of the blame for the situation grows. The child may grow into an adult whose perception of worth is always low and leads them into self-destructive situations and unequal relationships.

These harmful influences have been well-documented in situations where physical violence of a non-sexual nature has been recognized, and it is being gradually realized that, in many cases, sexual abuse is but one variation of physical abuse.

COPING WITH SEXUAL AROUSAL

The disclosure of enjoyment as part of the emotional response of the child is even more difficult to accept and discuss. It is enjoyable to be singled out for a 'special relationship' even if secret and hidden from the world. Even very small children masturbate and show signs of sexual excitement. It is impossible to be stimulated sexually without responding in some way, and the sexual excitement that is felt can be dealt with in a variety of ways.

Some children show behaviour which is regarded as precociously sexual. They have learnt to relate to adults only in a sexual way. In the surgery they lean against the doctor's leg and flirt provocatively, kissing the doctor on the lips in a suggestive way before they leave. (Foster parents or teachers may complain of more overt sexual overtures.) And how do the non-involved adults respond? Only too often by thoughts such as 'they must have asked for it'. The doctor feels uncomfortable being treated in this sexual way, and needs to recognize the feeling of sexual excitement in the room (not deny it, or blame the child who has learnt that this is the way to behave with adults).

Other children learn to cope with the emotional overload and confusion of roles by denial of any feeling: they become remote and inaccessible. They may fail to thrive and go on to show many of the features that we accept as pathognomic of physical abuse. Many others hide their feelings so well that it is only when a particular trigger in adult life makes them more vulnerable that the defences are lowered and the story emerges.

HELPING THE ADULT

The abused children grow into adults and it is with these that most general practitioners will be involved. Understanding how they have coped with their emotional feelings when children, can help when sexual abuse is disclosed in adult life.

Mrs M had made the first appointment on a Monday morning. She came in looking distraught and had been weeping. A month before she had been seen after a very early miscarriage at six weeks and had appeared disproportionately upset over the loss of what had been an unplanned pregnancy. This time, after much hesitation, hand-wringing and looking away from the doctor, she said that she and a friend had been talking about their parents. She had been telling her friend how strict her father had been when her friend said 'At least you weren't abused'. She had burst into tears and been unable to tell her friend any more. Her friend had persuaded her that she must confide in the doctor.

At this point in her story, she stopped and sought assurances from the doctor that nothing was going to be written down and that nothing would happen to the 'person involved'. When assured that nothing would happen unless someone was now at risk, she was able to reveal that it had been her father. She said that he had 'gone through a bad patch' when her parents were not getting on and used to come back home from the pub and get into bed with her. She described what had happened over several years in a flat voice with no emotion, as though it had happened to someone else.

'How do you feel about what happened?' asked the doctor. Mrs M changed the subject – she was sure he didn't really know what he was doing and sought to excuse him from blame. The doctor asked

'If he is not to blame, who is?' She sat, miserable, with tears running down her face. The doctor, unable to tolerate the despair, said 'You feel that it's your fault?' and as Mrs M nodded, sniffing, the doctor went on 'How old were you when it started?' 'I was in junior school, I must have been about nine.' Long silence. 'I suppose I couldn't really have stopped him, we always had to do what he said.' Mrs M was able to move on to accept that perhaps she was not responsible for what had happened and even to accept that her father must have known what he was doing, and remember episodes which indicated that he knew it was wrong and had to be concealed.

Mrs M had accepted the burden of guilt. She had been unable to blame her father whom she still loved and looked up to. Her position was still one of inequality and submissiveness.

It is noticeable that in the exchange above the doctor was led into direct authoritarian questioning as a result of the patient's attitude of helplessness and inferiority. A sharing of the anguish would have been a more appropriate and preferred means of proceeding in a more equal relationship. Attention to the doctor-patient interaction here gives clues as to how the patient views the world and relates to it from a particular stance, in this case a 'victim' stance. The doctor was able to remember how the patient had said of her miscarriage 'Everything always goes wrong for me'.

In a later consultation, Mrs M was talking again about the events of her childhood. In an astonished tone of voice she said 'When I was sitting on top of him and going up and down, I remember feeling warm, no hot, right up my body to my neck and face, and afterwards I would snuggle that warm feeling to myself right inside me and it kept me from minding when he was shouting and hitting me when I'd done something he thought was

> wrong. I'd forgotten about that.' She sat and thought about what she had said. The doctor noticed how flushed and excited she looked. It was difficult to remain quiet and not use words to flee from the moment of revelation of sexual feeling. Mrs M looked directly at the doctor and blushed even more. The doctor said quietly, so as not to disturb the atmosphere of excited complicity, 'It's a very powerful feeling, isn't it', and Mrs M looked relieved and her blush faded.

It would have been much more comfortable for the doctor to run away from this illicit sexual feeling. If this had been done the patient would have been confirmed in her ideas that these feelings were unnatural, abnormal, and in need of concealment and strict control. This would have delayed or even prevented her recognition of her emotions as normal sexual responsiveness. Her difficulties in responding to her husband's sexual approaches would have continued. Having shared with the doctor the knowledge that these feelings were so powerful, Mrs M was able to go on to recognize and own her sexual feelings as normal and healthy despite the circumstances in which they were first aroused. (A follow-up consultation with Mrs M is reported in Chapter 11.)

The strength of the emotions of guilt and sexual excitement tend to make the doctor behave in a defensive and evasive way in order to avoid confrontation with these dangerous areas. However, if avoided, the guilt cannot be examined for its origins in the powerlessness of the exploited child. Defensive avoidance will also prevent the doctor from being able to trace the excitement to its sources in normal sexual responsiveness whatever the circumstances, and in the forbidden nature of the experience.

Recognition that these feelings may be present can prompt the doctor into probing the defences prematurely to identify the guilt and excitement. If the patient is not ready to accept these powerful feelings, attempting to force the pace will result in continued denial that they exist. Asking questions to elicit the feelings invites refutation. Patients need to find their own way back to remembered feelings that the doctor cannot know about. Only then can they be acknowledged and accepted.

6

Deeper troubles

So far we have looked at problems presented by patients in primary care which most doctors would recognize as being within the primary care remit. Patients present in surgery and the doctor does not have any idea what is expected from the consultation until it unfolds. It is not possible to avoid encounters with patients who have queries about normal sexual feelings in parent-child interactions, who have sexual difficulties, or who have complaints of present or prior sexual abuse.

Some doctors will prefer to refer these patients on to other sources of help (where they exist and when the patient will agree). Sexual abuse therapy groups, clinical psychologists, community psychiatric nurses, rape crisis centres, sexual therapy clinics, and psychiatrists all have such patients in their case loads. It may be possible to make an intra-practice referral to another member of a group practice who is more interested in this type of problem.

It is not so difficult for the doctor who has had some training to cope with presentations of this nature. Seminar training with the Institute of Psychosexual Medicine is particularly suitable for doctors in primary care. It concentrates on examining the interaction between the patient and the doctor in order to interpret to the patient how he or she interacts with others. Developed from Balint training, it enables doctors to become at ease discussing sexual matters, to understand their own bias, and to use the doctor-patient relationship in a therapeutic way. But even for doctors who have received this seminar training it may not be easy to 'hear' the underlying problem.

THE INDEX OF SUSPICION

What factors might raise the index of suspicion that sexual abuse might be germane to problems experienced by patients? Prior sexual abuse has been implicated in the causation of a multiplicity of conditions. Schei and Bakketeig (1989) looked at a random sample of women in the city of Trondheim. They found that a history of physical or sexual abuse was associated with sexual problems in the current or previous relationships of these women as well as the occurrence of a higher incidence of gynaecological symptoms. Common psychological problems found are eating disorders, depression, agoraphobia, relationship problems and underlying low self-esteem (Jehu, 1988). Many of these problems are expressed as physical, somatized, complaints of ill-health. How many of the 'heart-sink' patients seen in general practice fall into these categories?

Patients who present in this way find it difficult to complain overtly about their inner discomfort and anguish. Some covert presentations have already been reported in earlier chapters. Others are even more difficult to unravel.

Mrs W Had asked for a home visit. She had moved into the area and had no notes. An unconcerned-looking husband showed the doctor into the bedroom, where Mrs W lay, looking pale, plump and pathetic. The husband left the doctor to it. She was in 'terrible agony' she explained with a little girl look. Her previous doctor had given her 'really strong painkillers' for it but she had run out; could she have some more? The doctor explained that there were no notes through yet; could Mrs W tell him more about the problem. He sat on the side of the bed while she summarized her history. She had obviously told it many times before and there was no emotion in the account. The doctor lost count of the number of operations and investigations she had had. Bit by bit her reproductive organs had been removed. She had had bariums, endoscopies, examinations under anaesthetic; on and on went the catalogue. Finally the story of this intractable 'terrible' abdominal pain was finished.

Trying to make sense of what he had heard, the doctor said 'It sounds as if everyone has been looking for something terrible inside you but they can't find it'. For a moment Mrs W looked vulnerable and open, then the little girl defences shuttered across and tears welled from her eyes. 'Please help me, doctor', she sobbed. Disarmed he agreed to repeat her previous pain killers and left. Later he discussed the patient with his partners, having felt dissatisfied with his management. His partners pointed out how he had been manipulated and he resolved to do better.

Over many months he tried without success to bypass Mrs W's established pattern of behaviour with doctors. Then one day he arrived at the house to find her quite distraught. Her adopted daughter was emigrating to Australia. Mrs W had persuaded her husband to move to be near her daughter and now her daughter was going to leave her again. She was furious but unable to understand it except as an abandonment. In her anguish she let her defences fall and told the doctor how everyone had always let her down. The story emerged of a childhood where her mother had worked long hours to support the family, her father had been at home disabled with a chronic chest complaint. She could not remember a time when she had not looked after all her father's needs, including his sexual ones, until his premature death when she was in her teens. She saw him as good and kind, but he had left her. Her mother had never given her any support. She had always had abdominal pain since childhood; it became worse after she married and she could never have intercourse because of the pain.

This patient illustrates how it is not just the sexual abuse which affects the child, but the context in which it occurs. The experience of being powerless and violated can result in manifold symptoms in adult life. This woman had become a 'victim'. The distortion of the relationships within this family had set up conflicts which she could not resolve. She had supplanted her mother in the relationship with her father and her mother was seen as absent and not supportive. The normal maturation processes were by-passed as she was forced into the role of the wife. She saw herself as having willingly accepted this role which she knew to be wrong; therefore it was her fault that it happened. She had no 'childhood' during which she could be dependent and trust the adults in her family, and as she became an adult she sought constantly to obtain this caring relationship from those around her. Her abdominal pain could be seen as an expression of her conflict and guilt. Her continuing search for the 'badness' within had manipulated doctors into inappropriate medical and surgical treatments. She felt that all the doctors had let her down as well; she depended on them as a child on its parents, to protect her from the 'badness', to root it out and rid her of it, and they had all failed her. She had chosen a mild and 'good' husband who had coped with her constant dependancy demands and somatic complaints by retreating into remote and distant behaviour. In turn she had attempted to lean on her adopted daughter who retreated physically as well as emotionally – the daughter was having to flee to Australia to escape.

Patients such as Mrs W frequently receive derogatory labels from their doctors. They are seen as 'hysterical' or 'neurotic', their attention-seeking and manipulative behaviour being viewed as an attempt to usurp the power of the medical profession. It is, however, their feeling of powerlessness that makes them manipulative – people with self-confidence can ask for things for themselves directly; those with a low self-esteem have to manoeuvre indirectly for they fear the repeated pain of rejection.

MORE HIDDEN PROBLEMS

K came into the surgery already on the brink of tears. She could not cope at work. She had had a row with the supervisor and had walked out.

As the halting story of all her problems emerged – her marriage was shaky, she was in financial difficulties – the doctor began to feel irritated. K was handing all of these problems over to the doctor. 'How can I help you?', the doctor asked. No answer was forthcoming; a catalogue of woe and numerous reasons why K could not do anything about any of her problems ensued. The doctor noted her own increasing anger but managed to recognize that the emotion was coming from the patient. She said 'You must get very frustrated about all these things that you feel you can't do anything about.' This released even more anger and the tears flowed with great heaving sobs. The doctor sat silent, trying to avoid actions which might be interpreted as a rejection or non-acceptance of this powerful emotional moment. When the flow eased, doctor and patient were able to negotiate more openly what would be practical and helpful to cope with the crisis, and the doctor offered to give the patient some time to try and sort out why everything seemed to be going wrong.

In subsequent consultations, an account of the background gradually emerged between the constant complaints. K was one of six children, her father had been an alcoholic and had 'knocked' her mother about. She also slipped in that he was 'strange'. The doctor missed this at first and had to return to it later. This proved very difficult; K was all too forthcoming about all her current problems and most of her upbringing, bombarding the doctor with too much information, but evasive on the subject of her father's 'strangeness'. Each time the doctor brought this into the consultation K would change tack and launch into some other disaster that had befallen her. Eventually the doctor managed to pin her down; K said 'Well, he used to make me touch him', and again tried to go off at a tangent. By then the doctor was sure that behind the defence lay an important piece of information, and had sufficient rapport to be able to point out to K what she was doing.

The story emerged that her father had got her to masturbate him, that this had progressed to fellatio, but he had never tried to stimulate or penetrate her. She said that he could not help it – it was the drink – and she had never tried to stop him because she had to protect her mother from his violence. She described vividly how, now, if she saw her husband's penis, she wanted to be sick and her heart pounded with fear and excitement. She could only make love in the dark and she could not touch the penis at all. Her husband had accused her of being frigid and not loving him.

This patient had considerable personality problems. She viewed everything that happened to her as outside her control. Her powerlessness and anger led to confused signals to her doctor, who became irritated and angry. Her alternating submissive or belligerent attitudes at work had led to her feeling exploited and to conflict with her supervisor.

Her inability to express her own needs and wishes directly, had led to arguments in her marriage. She felt responsible for what had happened between her and her father. Not only had she agreed to do it (to keep the peace) but she could admit to excitement while carrying out something which she was later aware was 'strange'. Her lack of power within the family situation made her vulnerable to exploitation, and her pattern of response carried on into adult life.

PATRIARCHAL POWER

Both these case histories illustrate types of families in which the father expects to be looked after, fed, comforted, obeyed and sexually satisfied. The fathers are often performing less well in the outside world; they may be ill, unemployed, in low status jobs or just feel inadequate compared with their peer group. Within the home it is a different story; their power is absolute. The power is not always shown overtly by physical or verbal dominance, patriarchal authority can be exercised by the rest of the family trying to 'keep the peace' and anticipate his wishes.

Children in these families are captive, totally dependent on the parents for their basic needs. There is often little contact with others outside the family group, with restrictions on any activities which might lead to social contact by wife or children. The limitations are presented as part of the 'caring' of the father to protect the members of the family from the aggression the father 'knows' is out there in the wider world (he knows it is there because he has it within himself). The fantasy about the dangers of the outside world has to be contrasted with the reality that the least safe place for women and children is within the home – most sexual abuse takes place in their own homes.

Weinberg (1955) classified abusers into three types and

these categories appear in much of the subsequent literature. The 'paedophile' appears to be the least common type, but the most often reported in the media and used to try to frighten women and children into remaining inside their own homes. These are described as the 'Strangers' who attack indiscriminately; who are attracted to places where children are likely to be found, such as parks or schools.

Most abusers from reported cases of sexual abuse fall into Weinberg's other categories. The 'endogamic' fathers are family-centred and do not want outside social contacts. Tormes (1972) describes these abusing men as affection-seeking, passive men who rule the household by keeping control of all the money and by being ill-tempered and over-protective. They appear to the outside world as caring family men who are constantly preoccupied with the family business and reduce the other members of the family to ciphers whose wishes count for nothing.

The other category described is the 'psychopathic' man. Later researchers found these abusers to be physically as well as sexually violent. Tormes found that these men were often ineffectual outside the home but tyrants within. Typically they are emotionally-dependent on their wives and children, suspicious of any extrafamilial contacts, and resorting to sexual abuse either as part of general physical violence or when the wife is sexually unavailable. Alcohol is sometimes used by these men and their families to excuse their lack of control. Most of the men in the latter two categories were respected by their peers and appeared quite normal until their behaviour within the home was exposed.

MOTHERS AND GRANDMOTHERS

The role of the mother has been discussed briefly in Chapter 3. Frequently the story of abuse includes the absence of the mother, physically or metaphorically. She was not there, did not protect the child, or did not see or hear what was happening.

Various theoretical explanations have been proposed to explain these disturbed family relationships. For instance, it has been suggested that because male children wish to possess their mothers, when they grow up to become fathers they identify their daughters as their mothers and wish to possess them in turn. Kaufman *et al.* (1954) suggested a three-generational theory – the maternal grandmothers were stern, demanding and cold, bringing up their families on their own. The grandfathers were absent due to death or abandonment. The grandmothers pampered their sons but expected their daughters to be strong and capable like themselves. These daughters in turn tried to make their own daughters (the granddaughters) into mothers to satisfy their own unmet childhood needs. The fathers of these girls became involved in incestuous activity with their daughters (the granddaughters) who had been made into little mothers. It has to be assumed that the grandmothers who seem so powerful and strong in raising their families also had unmet dependency needs which rendered them powerless to protect their granddaughters.

However, these generational theories do nothing to explain the incidence of anal abuse of sons.

If wives and children are regarded as possessions and patriarchal power is misused, sexual abuse becomes understandable as part of the spectrum of violence against weaker members of society. Historically, it is only just over one hundred years ago in Britain that married women were given the right to own their own property, or that a mother's custodial rights over her children have been recognized. In many other countries these same rights have yet to be attained.

THE CYCLE OF POWERLESSNESS

Children who are brought up in families isolated from other systems of social order will tend to continue the cycle of powerlessness when they have families of their own. It has been seen already that families in which sexual abuse occurs are often socially isolated and not in contact with alternative ways of functioning. If, within the family, children (and wives) have no rights over their own bodies, they can be used by those who have the authority over them.

Mrs W illustrates the sense of powerlessness being continued from childhood to adult life, crippling the ability to form equal relationships within the family, and with professionals who offer help. The cycle rotates to set the scene for another generation to be brought up in an environment where abuse is more likely. Intervention which enables the adult to understand and come to terms with the sense of powerlessness could break the cycle and have far-reaching benefits for the next generation of children and future parents.

REFERENCES

Jehu, D. (1988) *Beyond Sexual Abuse* John Wiley & Sons Ltd, Chichester.

Kaufman, I., Peck, A. and Tagivri, C. (1954) The Family Constellation and Overt Incestuous Relations between Father and Daughter. *American Journal of Orthopsychiatry*, **24**, 266–75.

Schei, B. and Bakketeig, L. S. (1989) Gynaecological impact of sexual and physical abuse by spouse. A study of a random sample of Norwegian women. *Br. J. Obstetrics & Gynaecology,* **96**, 1379–83.

Tormes, Y. (1972) *Child Victims of Incest*, American Humane Association Publication, Denver.

Weinberg, S. (1955) *Incest Behaviour*, Citadel Press, New York.

7

The chronic patient: damage limitation

Within any group of patients, there will be those who can be given very little help. All doctors have to come to terms with the knowledge that they cannot 'save the world' and that there is a limit to what can be done.

There are many illnesses that are ill-understood and for which there is no cure. This does not mean to say that the doctor should turn the patient away with curt words that nothing can be done. If nothing else, patients can be helped to accept the damaged state in which they find themselves. Just as with multiple sclerosis or renal failure where the damage is done and cannot be repaired, so too with very damaged personalities, a cure cannot be expected. After these patients have been 'examined' and found to be 'incurable' the specialist discharges them from follow-up and the general practitioner is left with having to continue to cope with their needs.

IRRITATING DEMANDS

The doctor felt irritated the moment R came in and moved her chair too close. R was well known to the whole practice. Mildly mentally handicapped she always managed to get the receptionists to 'fit her in' whenever she turned up. After an inappropriate social interchange (R always asked personal questions of the doctor which were fended off) she scrabbled around in the voluminous, rather battered, handbag and produced several sheets of paper torn from an exercise book. She announced, rather proudly, that she had written it all down. The doctor frowned and poked the sheets with a finger. (R looked excited and was obviously expecting something that the doctor suspected, from previous encounters, would be difficult or impossible to supply.) R explained that she had been watching 'that programme' and had decided that she must tell the doctor about what had happened to her before she was taken into care. The doctor found herself agreeing to read the sheets and see R 'next week'.

The doctor found it difficult to decipher some of the writing, but the meaning was clear. It was a catalogue of horrifying physical and sexual abuse in lurid detail. Was it true or the product of video nasties? The doctor went back through R's voluminous notes. There, from early on, was a case conference report that appeared to confirm the physical abuse, although there was no mention of sexual abuse. The doctor felt guilty for the impatience felt with this inadequate woman, unable to form proper relationships, and constantly making people feel uncomfortable with her inappropriate social overtures.

R, as usual turning up when she felt like it, saw other partners about various minor problems, but did not mention her script to them. When several weeks later, she saw the same doctor again, she came with a different problem. The doctor, tentatively, brought up the subject and asked if R wanted to talk about it. 'No, not today, thanks,' she remarked brightly, leaving the doctor feeling frustrated and, once again, irritated.

It was possible for these consultations to be discussed at a practice meeting and from this a better understanding was reached of the interaction between R and the various practice members. It could be understood and accepted that R, despite her adult years, behaved to the staff as though she were a child. They responded by feeling parental and protective and 'fitted her in' whenever she wanted. Her inept social interactions could be recognized as her attempt to copy the observed behaviour of social workers and care staff, after the vacuum left by her previous abusive relationships. No wonder the doctors had felt irritated – now they could recognize the patronizing or jolly tones of the care staff keeping their emotional distance. The insight gained by all the practice members helped them to cope better with this patient. Her inept social interactions which had previously prevented proper thought could be kept in proportion, and more constructive use made of the consultations. It is difficult to envisage how the early damage to this patient could be repaired. Her patterns of behaviour were well established and there was no reason for her to want to change.

THE BURDEN OF THE INCURABLE

Mr T was thin and grey-looking. He looked much older than his years, more like 50 than late-30s. He gave his obviously prepared history in a quiet, tired voice. He was a recovered alcoholic and had been recommended to this doctor by others in Alcoholics Anonymous. He said he had had experiences as a child which he felt he was now ready to deal with and would like some help to do this. Could the doctor spare some time to do this? (Already the doctor felt weighed down by the burden this patient was carrying.) Arrangements were made to set aside some longer consultations for this task.

Over the next few weeks, Mr T recounted his story of sexual abuse from his father and his uncle during the whole of his childhood. He had run away from home and been put into a children's home where abuse, this time from a staff member, had continued. He had progressed to crime, borstal, and then prison. Always his relationships had ended in buggery, and his alcohol intake was constant and excessive. Now dried out, he had a relationship 'of a sort' with another man, who was keen for him to learn to 'respond normally'. He remarked with considerable insight that all he felt for his friend was gratitude and this was a basis for future resentment and another relationship 'down the drain'.

The doctor remarked on several occasions about his lack of anger towards the perpetrators of his violations. Mr T said his anger was all used up; he had tried to destroy himself, knowing that he was worthless, but he couldn't even do that properly. He would have to go on living in this hell of a life. The doctor was overwhelmed and shared this with the patient – the support the patient produced for the doctor surprised them both and the first frost-bitten smile appeared on the face of the patient. Eventually, Mr T 'called it a day', thanking the doctor for 'making him feel like a human being with something to give', but acknowledging that the early damage made it impossible for him to respond 'normally' or to find a sexual response within himself.

This patient had gained significant skills of his own during prolonged contact with social workers, probation officers, and in Alcoholics Anonymous. He had considerable insight and little expectation of radical change. The help that was given was more in the nature of the 'befriending' to which he was accustomed but he had recognized that he needed someone outside that organization to be able to withstand such a burden. The acknowledgement that the burden was too great for the doctor to carry, enabled the patient to recognize his own strengths and to continue.

HOW EXTENSIVE IS THE DAMAGE?

It is impossible to quantify the number of people who remain undamaged by sexual abuse. By the nature of their work, psychiatrists, psychologists and medical staff dealing with ill people are bound to see those who have been damaged and few who have not. Many research papers have described the long-term consequences of sexual abuse, but it would be wrong to conclude that everybody who has these experiences suffers to the same degree or has the same long-term problems. The more severe end of this spectrum is described in Sheldon (1988); her article illustrates how the experience of being powerless, violated and betrayed by trusted figures can result in manifold symptoms in adult life. There may not be overt, disclosure of the previous abuse, especially in early interviews.

Briere (1984) defines a 'post-sexual abuse syndrome' which he compares closely to the criteria for 'borderline personality disorder'. Briere's definition includes dissociation, sleep disturbance and nightmares, anxiety attacks, feelings of isolation, chronic muscle tension, problems with anger, sexual dysfunction, parasuicide and self-mutilatory behaviour, alcohol and drug abuse, and repeated victimization in adult life.

In primary care a large number of the patients who fall into the 'frequent attender' category will exhibit some or all of these characteristics. Perhaps a greater awareness that these symptoms may have resulted from sexual abuse may make these patients easier for the doctor to understand and tolerate.

Unfortunately, the strong dependency needs, the testing

out of treatment boundaries, and the desires for an exclusive relationship with the doctor make these people difficult patients to tolerate for any length of time. The doctor must guard against providing a bottomless well of support which increases the dependency and powerlessness of the individual, enervates the doctor and limits the availability of the doctor for others.

REFERENCES

Briere, J. (1984) *The effects of childhood sexual abuse on later psychological functioning: defining a Post Sexual Abuse Syndrome*. Paper presented at the 3rd National Conference Sexual Victimisation of Children, Childrens Hospital National Medical Center, Washington DC.

Sheldon, H. (1988) Childhood Sexual Abuse in Adult Female Psychotherapy Referrals: Incidence and Implications for Treatment. *Br J. Psychiatry*, **152**, 107–11.

8

Action stations: dilemmas for the doctor

In some ways the presentation of current abuse might seem an easier task to deal with than prior abuse. There are carefully laid down procedures for dealing with current child sexual abuse which have to be followed (*Diagnosis of child sexual abuse*; Standing Medical Advisory Committee of the DHSS, 1988). The doctor of first contact does not want to become too involved, and must avoid the victim needing to repeat the allegations more than absolutely necessary.

Most child sexual abuse cases can and should be handled by existing child protection agencies. Every general practitioner has been supplied with a booklet outlining the procedures to be followed in their area. The Social Services Department has a legal duty to make enquiries and to take action whenever information suggesting child abuse is received. The NSPCC, the Police and paediatric specialists all have responsibilities and statutory duties. When a general practitioner is the person of first contact, care must be taken that vital evidence, both verbal and material, is not lost. Going over incidents may make future management more difficult.

The responsibility for sorting out what should be done is not the doctor's alone; co-operation with others can allow doctors to distance themselves to some extent from the acute problem. Avoidance of involvement in acute decisions can make the doctor appear less partisan to the patient and family, and a more acceptable source of help and advice in the future.

EFFECTS ON THE DOCTOR

But what effect does hearing such accounts have on the doctor? Coming to terms with one's own sexuality and potential to exploit can be difficult and may unearth repressed and painful feelings. The voyeurism and morbid excited interest that sexual advances towards children arouses in all of us needs to be recognized. The guilt of the victim may tempt the doctor into collusion that it is the fault of the victim. The anger of the one penetrated and damaged may produce violent reactions in the listener who cannot then hold to the therapeutic role and becomes an avenger on behalf of the helpless one.

Male doctors have the added difficulty of having to deal with the uncomfortable fact that 85–90% of abusers are male. They cannot identify with the abuser and cannot believe that men that they know could behave in this way. Therefore they conclude that the abuser must be abnormal. Similarly, female doctors identify with the maternal role and feel affronted and horrified by the lack of protection the child has received from the mother; they cannot, initially, understand how the mother failed to see what was happening. She, too, must be abnormal.

When physical abuse first became recognized, the adult was seen as evil and outside normality. As recognition of the problem became more widespread, the perpetrator could sometimes be recognized as a normal parent who momentarily lost control. With more compassion, programmes of prevention and rehabilitation became possible.

In cases involving sexual abuse, it is more difficult for

the public (which includes doctors!) to feel compassion for parents who cannot control their sexual impulses towards their children. But the needs of the child are very different from those of a society, excited and horrified by the nature of sexual abuse, and demanding retribution. The price of justice may be seen by the child as a punishment for speaking out. The child sees the family being torn apart, the father in prison and the mother short of money and devoid of friends and support.

Where the doctor in primary care has the greatest role is in being accessible. It is acceptable to go to the doctor and present your calling card of 'ill-health', or other problems seen as 'medical'. How much more difficult to seek help from an unknown social worker in an unfamiliar office, or to find the right moment to speak to a teacher, or youth worker who sees the child in a different role.

Sexual abuse disguised as somatic complaints are the commonest presentation in general practice. Examples such as amenorrhoea and intractable abdominal pain have already been described, as well as the presentation of mother and daughter together. The following case illustrates further some of the hazards and pitfalls in a joint mother and daughter consultation.

PROTECTING THE CHILD

M was brought to the surgery by her mother, who asked for her to be seen urgently. She was a tall nine-year-old girl who looked older but was dressed in frills with a bow in her permed hair. In a monotone, the mother said that M had been doing 'naughty things with boys' and 'all the neighbours know what a wicked girl she is'. Mother wanted the doctor to examine M to see if she was 'intact' down there. Hastily, the doctor distanced herself from the problem. Had anyone else been told? Oh, yes, the school knew all about it and the social worker had been to see them.

At this point, a phone call provided relief. One of this doctor's partners had been contacted by Social Services already. The doctor left the pair of them, the girl standing quite separately from the drooping mother, to find out more. The doctor returned to explain that a special appointment with a specialist had been arranged for the morning and it seemed unnecessary to examine M. The mother argued and the doctor found herself defending both herself and the girl from the anger. She offered to see the mother again afterwards but was relieved when she did not turn up. The story was heard at second hand from the case reports.

It emerged that M had been sexually abused at least since she was a small child, possibly since infancy. She had become a child who sexualized all her relationships and had become notorious in the neighbourhood for being willing to sell her body for gifts or money. The mother was furious with M when a male teacher, alarmed by the provocative sexuality of this child, had referred her to Social Services and M had 'spilt the beans'.

It was understandable that the mother resented the disclosure, and blamed M for the disruption to the family that was bound to follow. She could not accept that she had any part to play in preventing the abuse, nor was she able to see that her husband had any responsibility for the control of his sexual needs. All the blame was heaped upon M. After all, was she not promiscuous and pert, (not like her grey and bowed mother), doing these sexy, exciting things with everyone?

The doctor had felt very uncomfortable and, thinking about the feelings later, had realized that the mother's request covered a wish to punish the girl by subjecting her to an examination, and that to agree would have been to collude with the mother in an acceptance of M's guilt. The doctor had felt that M needed protection, not further assault!

What could the doctor have done if there had not been a phone call to give relief from the dilemma? What are the alternatives? One is to acquiesce with the mother's demand to examine the child. However, the child is in no position to give informed consent for her own examination. She has not the maturity to understand the implications and would not be autonomous in the presence of her mother. To separate the girl from the mother in order to attempt to obtain consent, would expose the doctor to possible charges of assault. It is unlikely in such a case that the mother would agree to be excluded, as the hidden agenda appears to be the punishment of the girl for her behaviour. To examine the girl under these circumstances would indeed be an assault. And yet some arrangements have to be made for her examination.

After listening to more of the story, it may be established that the child is at immediate risk. Urgent contact with a paediatrician (preferably one with a special interest in child abuse) with a view to admission for the protection of the child, is the next step. Similar urgent action needs to be taken if the sexual assault is recent enough for evidence still to be present. Forensic specimens should be taken by a police surgeon or other doctor with special training in the procedures required, and well-versed in the sympathetic and skilful handling of this difficult situation to prevent further emotional damage from these procedures.

If the situation is not one of immediate danger, then Social Services (there is an emergency number for out-of-hours calls in the handbook) or the NSPCC should be contacted and the parents informed that this is what has to be done.

THE BALANCE OF EVIDENCE

Child sexual abuse is a criminal offence. The allegations have to be corroborated by material evidence. In the case of a pre-verbal infant, evidence will necessarily have to be of a physical nature. Suspicions would have to be backed up by the presence of physical damage; the smaller the child, the larger the adult is by comparison and the more likely that forceable penetration of orifices will leave physical signs of damage. Suspicions may be raised if the doctor is asked for advice about a vaginal discharge, or vulval soreness, or bleeding from the back passage in a child. One doctor, trying to do his best for a small child with extensive perianal warts, enquired of the accompanying parents whether sexual abuse had crossed their minds as a possible cause. The doctor never discovered what the parents really thought as the violence of their reaction and immediate removal of the family from that doctor's care, precluded any further enquiry.

Where the condition raises any suspicions, referral to an experienced paediatrician for investigation is a wiser course than trying alone to establish the balance of evidence. In the most sensitive cases, or where levels of anxiety are high in the doctor or other adult, a telephone call or personal contact may be the best way to pass on the concern. Types of abuse occurring in small children where physical damage is not apparent will not be identifiable unless witnessed by an adult or by another older child who can verbalize clearly.

A judge may now direct a jury that someone can be convicted on the uncorroborated evidence of a child. In cases of suspected childhood abuse, this evidence may be the story obtained from the child by reliable witness. The value placed on this account is higher if it is obtained soon after the alleged abuse, and if the story contains elements that a small child is unlikely to know about otherwise, like the stickiness of semen. Evidence from more than one child is more likely to be believed, or if child-pornographic pictures are discovered.

In general, the younger the child, the less reliance is placed on verbal corroboration and the greater on signs of physical injury. Accurate assessment by an experienced police surgeon or paediatric specialist may be vital and early referral will be the child's best protection.

Reliance on one or two markers of abuse can be misleading. Even venereal disease is occasionally spread without sexual contact, and the dangers of using reflex anal dilatation as a single diagnostic test were well illustrated during the Cleveland enquiry (Butler-Sloss, 1988). Early referral allows for the collection of evidence over a period of time; just as one bruise is insufficient for evidence of physical battering, the repetition of bruising over months or years becomes more and more conclusive.

BOTH SEXES ARE AT RISK

The older child can give a verbal account of sexual touching, of sexual organs being exposed, of being shown pornographic material or of penetrative intercourse. It must be emphasized that whenever the other person involved is older or in any position of authority and expects the activity to lead to his or her sexual arousal, then this is exploitative and abusive for the child. The popular image of sexual abuse occurring in older children is that between the teenage daughter and her father. However, in the Mori poll conducted for Channel 4 in 1984, the incidence of such events was 12 % for girls and 8 % for boys (Baker and Duncan, 1984).

When the older male child presents with physical symptoms such as abdominal pain, disturbance of bowel habit, or psychological symptoms such as stealing, running away from home or disruptive behaviour, the index of suspicion is not as high as it should be. The general low self-esteem and the way in which they value themselves only within a sexual relationship, may lead to abused teenage boys becoming involved in similar exploitative buggery outside the home, sometimes for emotional closeness, sometimes for financial gain. Particularly if the teenage boys become involved in criminal activities such as theft, damage to property or violence to others, they are likely to end up in care or custody. The hierarchy of power within these systems and the dangers presented by a few disturbed custodians can make the continuance of abuse likely (as was illustrated by the case of Mr T in Chapter 7). A greater awareness of the risk to boys may allow identification of those abused before they become abandoned to a system in which the pattern can be continued.

If there is any possibility that the perpetrator of the abuse may repeat the activity with another victim, then there is a duty to prevent anyone else being damaged. The older the victim, the more this duty devolves onto the abused individual, but the doctor must bear in mind that many victims continue to suffer from their lack of power in relationship to the rest of the world and may be unable to take independent action. For example, a woman revealed that she had been assaulted on many occasions by her brother. This brother had recently been deserted by his wife and was looking after the children. Social workers were already involved with the family and it might be necessary to contact them to give them this important information. In this case the abuse was long ago and it is difficult for the doctor to know the degree of current risk.

Children brought up in families where they are physically assaulted tend to repeat the pattern with their own families, but there is insufficient evidence about sexual assault to know if this, too, is repeated down the generations.

Doctors will not wish to be seen to be too suspicious and to be making accusations which cannot later be verified. However, the imbalance of power between children and their parents makes it imperative that other adults use their influence on the side of the child when he or she may be at risk. Because they are so vulnerable, their protection may become a duty which can override even that responsibility to the patient which is normally the primary concern of the physician.

WHEN ALL THE FAMILY ARE PATIENTS

After a child is referred with suspicion of abuse, the general practitioner will continue to have the members of the family as patients. The tasks here will be a combination of not interfering with the work of the other professionals involved, while still being seen as a supportive and accepting doctor. The doctor needs to guard against becoming a champion for one individual within the family, over-identifying with that person and colluding in manipulative behaviour.

> Mr G wept, his body shaken by his misery. His granddaughter had told her brother that Mr G had put his hand inside her pants and stroked her. Mr G's daughter (the child's mother) had confronted him after she had been informed about the episode and told him he must see the doctor, he must be 'ill'. He reminded the doctor about his awful wife, totally obsessed with her hypochondria, who had not responded to his needs, sexual or emotional, for many years. He said that his granddaughter had such a lovely soft body and she was such an affectionate child that he had got carried away with stroking her. The doctor felt sorry for this pathetic figure and almost fell into the trap of heaping the blame on the eight-year-old girl who had so 'seduced' him. Only a recognition of the feeling of colluding with Mr G to avoid attributing any 'nastiness' to this nice old man, saved the moment.

The general practitioner knew this family well and was able to ring Mr G's daughter.

If the daughter had not known about the abuse and if the doctor had not known her, a more formal approach either personally or via Social Services would have had to be made. Mr G would have to be informed that this was to be done, preferably with his consent. However, the confession implied that he wished to be stopped and was asking for external controls to be put on his behaviour. His guilty feelings enabled him to accept the need for others to know as part of the punishment he felt he deserved for his actions. (Even if consent was not obtained the need to protect the child must remain the priority.)

After discussion with the daughter and granddaughter as well, they decided that they would prefer to go to the Psychiatric Day Hospital for family therapy. The general practitioner was able to continue to see the members of the family for their medical needs (and there were an increased number of somatisized complaints presented during this time). The doctor had to deal tolerantly with these demands, understanding their origins, while remaining in touch with the progress of the therapy.

ETHICAL AND TECHNICAL DILEMMAS

The above illustrations are only some of the dilemmas presented by sexual violence. The types of quandaries fall into two main categories. Those involving the technical evidence are the easier to analyse. The more evidence, verbal and physical, the more the doctor can be certain about the existence of the assault. Where the symptoms and signs are sparse, reliance on one or two pieces of evidence may lead to false conclusions. The emotional impact of the suspicion of abuse must not be allowed to cloud the judgement when weighing up the technical indications.

The ethical dilemmas are more difficult. Doctors have little training in the examination of such difficulties and need to seek help, not only from colleagues, but also from other disciplines. It would be arrogant to assume that, because doctors have to deal with the results of sexual abuse, they have any better understanding of the ethical issues than anyone else.

For example, the removal of the violated child or the abuser from the family home may protect the child from further abuse but at what cost in the disruption of the family system? The child may be damaged in other ways by the loss of the father emotionally and physically, the family may become unsupported financially, with all that that entails, and the child may bear a greater burden of guilt for the damage done to all the family members.

Ethical issues like this need to be continually discussed and re-evaluated in the light of changing circumstances and attitudes. Although general practitioners may be the point of first contact, they must remain in contact with the other professionals involved in the care of the abused and with the changing social attitudes to the offence.

REFERENCES

Baker, A. W. and Duncan, S. P. (1985) Child Sexual Abuse – a study of prevalence in GB. *Child Abuse & Neglect*, **9**, 457–67.

Butler-Sloss, E. (1988) *Report of the enquiry into child abuse in Cleveland, 1987*, HMSO, London.

Standing Medical Advisory Committee of the DHSS (1988) *Diagnosis of Child Sexual Abuse: Guidance for doctors*, HMSO, London.

9

Rape

MYTHS AND MISUNDERSTANDINGS

Violent sexual abuse of children and rape have much in common. The perpetrator is in a position of power compared with the victim. Thus, just as the child is abused by the parent, older sibling, or other adult, so the female who is raped is subjugated by masculine strength and fear of further injury or death.

Women and children are still regarded by many, and often in law, as possessions of men. For instance, in England, until 1990 the law still followed the guidelines from 1736 that 'the husband cannot be guilty of rape committed by himself upon his lawful wife, for by their mutual consent and contract, the wife has given herself up in this kind to her husband, which she cannot retract.' In 1980, the Supreme Court in Israel abolished the husband's immunity saying 'English common law holds that a woman must submit herself totally to her husband. This is an outrage to human conscience and reason in an enlightened country in our time.'

Media reports about rape are always more indignant if the woman is violated by a man other than her husband, or if the woman is not yet married and not sexually experienced. There is frequently much less sense of outrage if the woman is a prostitute, or divorced, or single and sexually experienced – almost as though it is the violation of the man's property (wife or daughter) that is shocking, not the violation of the woman herself.

There are as many myths about rape as there are about childhood sexual abuse. It is widely believed that women have enjoyable fantasies about rape. Many men have misconceptions about women's fantasies, and they have difficulty in accepting that women do not necessarily want to act out any fantasies they may have. Fantasies about being chased or forced may come from deep within the woman's subconscious and may be enjoyable and erotic. The reality is very different. Rape is not enjoyable; it is degrading, frightening and vile.

In recently published surveys of *She* magazine readers, most of the men believed women enjoyed bondage whereas almost all the woman reported that they did not enjoy even the thought of this type of subjection. There are large numbers of jokes about rape which hide the reality of what it involves. Rape is a crime of violence. The Lord Justice General of Scotland said recently 'rape is an aggravated form of assault'. It can involve beating, physical restraint, the use of weapons, urinating or defecating and other forms of humiliation. Women are usually afraid that they will be killed and often continue to fear that this threat will be carried out after the event if they divulge what has happened. The fear and degradation are paralleled in childhood sexual abuse.

Another widely-held myth is that rape is committed by maniacs. This is similar to the belief that those who assault children physically or sexually are abnormal and can be recognized as such. In most cases of rape or child abuse the perpetrator is known to the victim. Similarly it is commonly believed that only certain types of women are raped and that the rapist is in the grip of an uncontrollable sexual urge. However, it can be shown that most rapes are planned and only occur when the situation is favourable for the man. If his urges were uncontrollable, he would not be able to suppress them, if, for instance, his plans were interrupted or altered by the unexpected presence of other people. The statistics from the London Rape Crisis Centre (1984) showed that in over 50 % of reported rapes the assailant was known to the woman, and that 60 % were raped inside a building, 30 % in their own homes. In childhood sexual abuse, almost all the perpetrators are known to the child and it frequently occurs in their own home.

REACTIONS TO RAPE

The reactions to rape are very similar to the sequelae observed in childhood sexual abuse sufferers. Burgess and Holmstrom (1974) identified what they described as the 'Rape Trauma Syndrome'. There is an initial acute phase in which physical symptoms predominate. These consist of the injuries sustained in the assault and the physical manifestations of the anxiety. They include muscle tension, sleep disturbance, gastrointestinal irritability with pain, anorexia and nausea, plus the genito-urinary symptoms of vaginal discharge, cystitis and pelvic pain, or rectal pain and bleeding.

In the second phase the woman reorganizes her life. She may move to a different part of the country, or turn to her family for support; she may develop fear of places which remind her of the location of the assault. Sexual fears emerge and sexual relationships may be severely affected. The woman during this stage appears outwardly well-adjusted, carrying on with normal activities, but there is denial and little interest in gaining insight.

In the third phase, or 'resolution', most women become depressed and need to talk. Anxieties present in the first stage reappear. This phase may be triggered by a court appearance where the woman often feels she is the one on trial. Particularly if the man is not convicted or has a trivial sentence, there is the guilt of feeling responsible for what has happened and the fear of another attack. Those who did not resist at the time of the rape seem most likely to be seriously troubled by their role in the rape, and to have thoughts that they could have prevented it if they had struggled. After the rape the women found it difficult to function as independent individuals with control over their own lives (McCrombie, 1975).

Compare this with the pattern of symptoms shown by childhood abuse victims. The youngsters may show various physical indicators such as difficulty with passage of urine or bowel movement, or be anxious or unhappy during toileting or nappy changing. There may be vaginal or anal discharge with stains on the underwear, together with pain or soreness. Oral soreness or discomfort may be present, and there may be other physical manifestations of assault. There is often sleep disturbance, abdominal pain, changes in appetite and anxiety symptoms. (Hobbs and Wynne, 1987). This corresponds almost exactly with the first stage of the Rape Trauma Syndrome described above.

The later stages of the Rape Trauma Syndrome are mirrored in the descriptions of the 'incest survivors symptoms' (Edwards and Donaldson, 1989) which include sexual and relationship problems, depression, self-esteem deficits, communication difficulties, self-destructive behaviour, feelings of shame or guilt as well as anger and hostility.

THE SENSE OF RESPONSIBILITY

T's mother attended her general practitioner to explain the problem. She was defensive and anxious to make clear that no blame attached to her. T still lived at home but at 19-years-old lived her own life, coming and going more or less as she pleased. She had gone to a local night-club about two months previously and she and a friend had met up with some boys they knew slightly. Her friend went off with one of the lads, leaving T with the other three. They had offered her a lift home but on the way, stopped and raped her. They drove back into town and threw her out. Fortunately for T, a woman was looking out of her window as this happened and when she saw T lying at the side of the road, called the police. Now after two months, the mother was anxious because T showed no signs of 'getting over it all'. The doctor suggested that T would be welcome to attend.

T was dressed in a shapeless sweater and baggy tracksuit bottoms, she was wearing no make-up and looked scrubbed clean. She looked unattractive and subdued. She said that she did not really want to talk about what had happened but her mother thought she should. She just wanted to forget about it. Everyone wanted her to go to court – the police, her parents and her friends – to have the boys punished. She had been thinking of getting a job somewhere else but couldn't think how to start. She had lost her job because she had not been to work for two weeks after 'that' had happened and she had got the sack. No, she had not told them at work why she had not gone to work. All this was recounted in a dull flat voice.

The doctor recognized that T felt responsible for what had happened and shared this with her. They went through the occurrences on that night and slowly T began to sit up straighter and look less submissive. T began to consider the possibility that it was not her fault that these boys had behaved like that; that she had not 'asked for it' by going to a night-club or by accepting a lift home with three lads that she knew, that she did not need to be punished further by losing her job.

Over the next few sessions T was able to come to terms with her inability to plan for her future, her need to wash and change into clean clothes several times a day, her fear about going out (and perhaps seeing the boys involved) and her feeling that everyone could see that she had been despoiled.

Her anger at what had happened spilled over and she had to recognize that it was just as inappropriate to blame her parents for 'letting her do what she wanted' as to accuse the night-club owners for 'letting people like that in'.

She was put in touch with a rape crisis centre who continued to help and support her, now that she could accept the need for assistance. She did decide to go ahead with being a witness for the prosecution but found this extremely distressing – 'almost as bad as the rape' she said – both because of the recollections required and because the insinuations of the defence counsel were so offensive (despite her preparations for the ordeal).

Initially T could deal with her ordeal only by trying to ignore it. She became depressed and unable to take decisions. She washed frequently and tried to look as sexless as possible. Once she understood why she felt like that she could begin to release the anger she felt, and she could release it with someone who was not involved and could recognize the inappropriate targets of her anger for what they were. She could gradually assume control over her own life again and decide for herself what she wanted to do. The doctor had to resist the tendency to take over the control, to avoid reinforcing her sense of helplessness, and at the same time be prepared to withstand the anger and show that it could be exposed without damaging either the doctor or patient.

It was important for the doctor not to be judgemental and to avoid any suggestions that might have compounded the guilt. The interactions are similar to those after any loss. With rape, there is a loss of control, a loss of the integrity of the individual, a sense of impotent, helpless rage and anger.

Those most affected by childhood sexual abuse and who exhibit the damaged personalities already outlined in earlier chapters, are also at more risk of rape as part of the general exploitation to which they have become accustomed. They do not know how to protest against it, nor do they understand that they should. Their guilt and low self-esteem for having been despoiled and violated prevents them from protecting themselves in the future.

RELEASING THE ANGER

One of the most important factors in recovering from sexual abuse is to be able to talk about what has happened. The victim may feel worthless and unable to ask for help because of a lack of self-esteem ('why should anyone want to listen to me?') or disbelief that it has happened (as in any disaster). They may become so angry that listeners, unless trained, cannot tolerate the emotions expressed.

Referral to a rape crisis centre is very helpful. Although rape crisis centres vary, most are run by women for women and provide an environment where the victim can control what contact she has, and can take what she needs – from just information on the telephone to full non-judgemental support in a group or by a trained individual. Those who become severely affected and need more specialist services can be referred for individual help from clinical psychologists, psychiatrists, or sexual therapy clinics as appropriate. The support from a rape crisis centre can include referrals to lawyers, or specialized housing agencies, and the individual contact can accompany the victim to police stations, courts and clinics if required.

Similar provision is beginning to be available for victims of childhood rape. Again this is biased towards helping women. The realization that male children and men are also subjected to rape is only just dawning; in some ways the loss of power and self-esteem is even more difficult to acknowledge. The abuse of males is still in the denial phase described earlier; its incidence is therefore unknown.

It is important for victims not to feel that they are being taken over but to know that they have autonomy and can ask for what help they require when they need it.

REFERENCES

Burgess, A. and Holmstrom, L. (1974) Rape Trauma Syndrome. *Am. J. Psychiat.*, **131**, 981–6.

Edwards, P. W. and Donaldson, M. A. (1989) Assessment of Symptoms in Adult Survivors of Incest. *Child Abuse & Neglect.*, **13**, 101–10.

Hobbs, C. J. and Wynne, J. M. (1987) Management of sexual abuse. *Arch. Disease in Childhood*, **62**, 1182–7.

The London Rape Crisis Centre *Sexual Violence*, (1984). The Women's Press Ltd, London.

McCrombie, S. (1975) *Characteristics of rape victims seen in crisis intervention*, The Rape Crisis Centre, PO Box 69, London WC1X 9NJ.

10

The doctor, the family and other professionals

Doctors are faced with having to deal, not only with those directly involved in sexual abuse, but also with those affected indirectly. The relatives of those involved, the teacher in whom the child first confides, the nurse who sees a father behaving in what seems an over-sexual manner to his daughter, the health visitor who has been visiting the family, friends of the family, other medical attendants, all of these have their own difficulties which they may wish to discuss with a skilful, listening doctor who can tolerate explicit sexual material. The immediate family are usually well catered for by the system set up to help the child and its parents, but other relatives have problems of their own.

THE ANXIETIES OF RELATIVES

Mr D attended the doctor with complaints of being tired all the time. There were no specific findings on examination or after some screening investigations. He was encouraged to look again at events that had happened since he had last felt well, to discover precipitating possibilities. He was able to

> talk to the doctor about his brother, who had been accused of rape. He had always rather admired his younger brother who worked in the same factory as himself. His brother was 'always a bit of a lad', played football well, had lots of mates at the pub and always seemed to be having a good time. His brother had been accused of forcing a girl (who worked in the office at the factory) to have intercourse with him when he gave her a lift home after seeing her waiting for a bus in the rain. Mr D's wife had said 'she must have asked for it' and he had been very angry with her for saying this. This girl was 'not like that', she was a young, innocent sort of lass, who talked to all the blokes at work without any of the snootiness that most of the office staff adopted. 'She didn't flirt with them neither, just talked like a human being.' Since then, he had felt very awkward with his brother, trying to avoid seeing him. He had gone off wanting sex with his wife, or even touching her, and she did not seem to mind. Mr D did not want to have any long appointments to sort out his problems; dealing with one feeling or difficulty was all he could cope with at a time.
>
> Over the following few weeks, during a number of brief appointments in surgery, he was able to realize how attracted he had been to this girl, and his ambivalent feelings of wishing to protect her and have her for himself. He could recognize that his wife had picked up some of his feelings and that she might feel some jealousy. He found it most difficult to reconcile his admiration for his brother for his 'male' behaviour with his condemnation when he 'went too far'.

Mr D had a picture in his mind of the sort of man who raped women. That sort was a monster, not normal, not like him, not like his brother. And yet, because he had known the girl, he believed her story – and because he knew his brother, he could believe he had behaved like that, despite admiring him for the manly attributes he felt his brother had in greater degree than most.

The myths about rape – that the woman asks for it by behaving in a certain way, that it is only certain types of women who are raped, that women lie about being forced, that it is committed by a maniac, or by someone who is overcome by uncontrollable sexual urges – all these came up against the reality of knowing both the people involved. At one point Mr D said, with great anguish, 'How can L (the girl) live in this awful world if she can't even have a lift home in the rain without being done up by an ordinary bloke like my brother?'. Mr D became very anxious that he, too, might damage a woman because he did not control himself. He became anxious that his wife might become someone else's victim and wanted her to stop work and only go out with him.

Neither he, nor his wife, were directly involved in the rape, but it had an enormous effect on them, on their relationship and eventually on how they both viewed the ways in which men and women should treat each other.

THE CONFLICTS FOR PROFESSIONALS

It is not just members of families who are affected by the contact with sexual abuse, but also the professionals who meet it in the course of their everyday work.

A nurse on a children's ward noticed that one girl's father leant over the bed and gave the girl open-mouthed kisses. She felt that this was not normal fatherly behaviour and reported her suspicions. Then the nurse had to cope with much the same reaction that a child or woman does on disclosure of sexual abuse. That she was taken seriously is a measure of how much more acceptable it is to have such suspicions nowadays. She was still made to feel, by many people, that it was her prim standards that were at fault, or that she should not have created all the anguish for the family who had to face an investigation.

She found that she was defending herself and saying that she was not prudish. She found it difficult to relate to her boyfriend in the same way as before. She wanted to show everyone that she had no sexual inhibitions but felt constrained by the maleness of her boyfriend – would he behave in an unacceptable and exploitative way also? There was a conflict between not telling anyone and possibly leaving the girl to be exploited by her father, and the observed distress of the whole family, including the girl, as these allegations were discussed.

The nurse needed to work through these feelings. No support was offered at work and she was made to feel inadequate for asking if she could talk it over with someone. She sought help from her general practitioner who saw her on a few occasions and helped her to come to terms with what she had to do.

THE NEED FOR AN UNSHOCKABLE DOCTOR

A doctor who worked as a school medical officer as well as in family planning clinics was rung up by a teacher desperately wanting to talk to someone. The teacher had been the first confidant of a child who had, after many years, told of abuse by a grandfather who lived with the family. The teacher perceived this particular doctor as being able to cope with talking about these sexual things because she did a family planning clinic.

Having passed on her information through the correct channels, the teacher had lost contact with the child who had been put into care. This had made her feel frustrated at not knowing the outcome, whether it had been 'the right thing' to do, and frustrated at her inability to continue the caring role she had adopted. Her doubts had arisen from knowing that the child would have to cope with the distress of telling her story again, and of being separated from her family, friends, and school.

The other predominant emotion that came across was that of excitement – partly due to the fact that the teacher herself had been the prime mover in a drama, but also excitement about the sexual content of what the girl had told her. The teacher had had to play this down when talking to colleagues – as she remarked, 'You can't go into detail about what happened between a child and her grandfather without shocking someone'.

The teacher had to sort out her own feelings; the sense of being a voyeur, the excitement of knowing about things that are forbidden, the sense of being shocked by the revelations but at the same time being titillated. The doctor had to be a very safe, unshockable, unaroused listener – and it was difficult to maintain this role in the face of all this stimulating material.

REFLECTED ANGER AND GUILT

As well as excitement about the sexual content of rape, or child sexual abuse, there are other emotions which may seem inappropriate to those on the periphery. For example, anger is frequently expressed.

> A doctor, on hearing that a grandmother had accused her son-in-law of abusing her grandchild, said 'I could kill that woman, she's always making trouble!'
>
> In another incident, the health visitor uncharacteristically exploded with 'They should whip him!', when she heard than an estranged husband had broken into the house and assaulted 'one of my mothers'.

It is interesting to note that the anger is often not directed at the perpetrator. The anger may be at the victim. One doctor said of an abused child 'No-one could possibly like her, she always leans on you and makes sexual advances, none of the teachers will be left alone with her for fear of what she might do'. How can these adults be frightened of what an 11-year-old can do? Similarly, a woman who has been raped can be subjected to derogatory insinuations to diminish her, or the mother of an abused child is often blamed angrily for not protecting the child. Where does all this anger come from? Is it inherent in the situation where one powerful person imposes their will to gain selfish sexual satisfaction? Does it, in fact, represent the anger of the perpetrator?

Guilt over failure to protect an assaulted child or woman may cause endless ruminations. 'If only I had gone home with her.' 'If only I had realized what was happening earlier.' This is often accompanied by an attempt to take over the running of someone's life – but the attacks have already made the victim feel out of control – the last thing they need is to hand over what little power remains. Those on the sidelines often try to make those directly affected deny that they still feel disturbed by what has happened. They will say 'Surely she should be over it by now?'.

TIME FOR REPAIR

It is difficult for those on the periphery to understand the global damage that is done to the victims. The range of disabilities from powerlessness, through vulnerability and isolation, to emotional control and numbness has been detailed in earlier chapters. Learning to revalue your own body and learning that it is possible to have control over how it is used is not a rapid process.

Similarly, those touched by contact with the victims need to have time to come to terms with the conflict between the myths and the reality of the abuse. General practitioners encounter such people not just as patients but also amongst their professional and social contacts. Doctors are viewed as suitable bulwarks to provide support, help and understanding. Sometimes the best course of action will be to direct them to other sources of help where a proper professional relationship can be maintained more easily. Where a doctor suspects that the experience at work may have acted as a trigger to expose hidden personal problems, referral is particularly necessary.

11

Edging forward

THE AFTERMATH

Some patients have coped with their experiences of sexual abuse already. During the course of examining other problems, the history of abuse will be mentioned almost in passing. It has already been shown (Chapter 4) that to focus on these events when they are not perceived by the patient as important, is unhelpful and misleading. It is often difficult to recall patients who give this type of history; because it is unimportant to them it is not recalled by the doctor as an integral part of the pattern of presentation.

Commonly, the experience of abuse happened on only one occasion and not within the enclosed family. For example, the perpetrator may have been a baby-sitter, or an uncle who was visiting and not well known. The victim tended to have a secure and emotionally supportive home life where sexual matters could be talked about openly. The episode was talked about and the victim's account believed. Action was taken to prevent a recurrence. The memory faded and became unimportant and was only remembered as another episode of distress that belonged in the past.

Other patients learn to come to terms with more traumatic

events. Repeated abuse, performed by someone such as a parent, who should be in a position of trust, and linked with threats which produced long-lasting fear and silence, is more likely to have caused deeper scars.

The research seminar on childhood sexual abuse reported at the scientific meeting of the Institute of Psychosexual Medicine in 1988, presented some preliminary findings from an examination of the cases presented to them. (Peebles *et al.*, 1988). They concluded that sexual abuse was often only a part of a childhood that was emotionally and physically deprived. The events surrounding the disclosure could affect the outcome and might be damaging in themselves. The long-term effects were more varied than would have been expected – they did not necessarily correspond with the nature or degree of the abuse.

These facets – the general family framework, the type, frequency and time span of the abuse, together with the reactions and events surrounding and following the discovery of the abuse, all affect the outcome and must be considered for each individual. Sexual abuse has tended to be viewed in isolation but the framework in which it occurs needs to be studied in order to make sense of the damage to the individual.

Much more work on the outcome needs to be done. For example, if the effects of the events at the time of disclosure could be better understood, rational changes in procedures could be made to prevent further emotional damage occurring.

OPTIONS FOR TREATMENT

When sexual abuse is uncovered the options for treatment depend on many factors. Firstly the patient may not wish to have any intervention. If no-one else is at risk, then no action need be taken, except to leave the patient aware that help is available if required. Hooper (1990) sent a questionnaire about sexual abuse in childhood to all his patients between 20 and 60 years of age. Replies were received from 418 patients (65 %) and of these 14 % admitted experiencing sexual abuse as a child. Despite this, only one patient took up the offer of counselling.

If the patient does seek help, this can be offered at several different levels. It may be within the competence of the individual general practitioner to offer help. The work is difficult and demanding and is not for everyone. Specific skills for dealing with psychosexual problems, such as those gained during seminar training with the Institute of Psychosexual Medicine (11 Chandos St, Cavendish Square, London W1M 9DE) may help the doctor tolerate the distressing nature of the complaint, talk more easily about sexual matters, and help the patient come to terms with what has occurred.

> Mrs M was reported in Chapter 5. After three consultations she said that she did not want a further appointment. She felt that she did not want to look at this problem anymore. She had managed to tell her husband a little about her childhood experiences; he had responded with anger against her father and had said that she was not to visit him again. She said 'I told him I couldn't do that, poor old man, he hasn't got anyone now who cares for him at all'. She could see that her own anger and terror of this powerful figure from her childhood had, to some degree, faded; she could pity him instead. She accepted the interpretation from the doctor that she felt she had to stand up for herself now. She accepted gracefully the offer from the doctor to re-attend if she thought it would be helpful.

Mrs M was going to have to work out a different relationship with her father. Up to now she had visited him fearfully. Her new feelings of self-confidence made her want to find a better way by herself. She could even disagree with her husband's suggestion of how she could cope with her father in the future.

> Mrs M was seen again several weeks later for a routine contraceptive check. She said she had decided not to have a baby just yet; as she put it about her husband – 'He's finding the new me a bit difficult to cope with and I think we've got some sorting out to do before a baby comes on the scene!'. She told the doctor that she had talked to her father and made arrangements for him to have some help with his washing and cleaning. That way she would not feel that she had to do it and she would not feel guilty about neglecting him. She said his health was really getting very bad but her mother would have nothing to do with him now. Her brother had said 'It serves the b . . . right!'. She said that her father had tried to bully her into saying she would visit him every day to do his shopping and anything else that needed doing, but she had told him that she had a life of her own to run. With a wry smile she said, 'You know, I do love him in a funny kind of way, but I don't like him much and neither does anyone else! Poor old chap, people just can't get on with him at all – he's always telling people what to do and when they stand up to him he goes all whining and pathetic – ever so irritating!'.

Mrs M would not be able to forget what had happened to her. It is likely that she and her husband will have to make some adjustments to their relationship now that she has become more self-confident and assertive. If she does decide to have a baby this may be a trigger for more of her feelings to come to the surface. She may require further help when any life change challenges her new-found sense of autonomy. For the time being she has resolved her feelings towards her father and has accepted what happened as being part of her past, rather than letting it affect her current everyday relationships.

One of the advantages of help being offered in primary care is the continuing availability of the general practitioner. It is unlikely that total acceptance or reconciliation with the abuser is possible, but the availability of a trusted doctor whom the patient can contact easily provides an opportunity for continuing therapy. The conflicting emotions can be re-examined at different periods throughout life, particularly at moments such as new relationships, childbirth, or death of a parent.

Patients can take the opportunity afforded during consultations to broach the subject again. A new crisis may bring the problem to the fore, enabling further work to be done and providing an opportunity for the patient to edge forward in recognition and resolution of the damaging events.

Many doctors will not wish to be involved in therapy, or are aware that they lack the skills to help the patient. Referral may also be preferable for those patients who do not want their general practitioner to know too much about them, or who wish their physical and emotional problems to be treated separately. A psychosexual problems clinic, individual psychotherapy, group psychotherapy, treatment by a clinical psychologist or full psychoanalysis are all possibilities which can be explored.

In Chapter 7 some patients were described who had been so damaged by their experiences that little could be done to help them. It is unrealistic to believe that all patients seeking help can or should receive treatment. Such patients may be helped to come to terms with their disability, but the doctor should not strive for impossible changes. General support from self-help groups, or where there are more specific difficulties, from social workers, health visitors and other professionals may be more genuinely useful than an illusion of radical reversal of the damage sustained.

THE SPECIAL NEEDS OF THE ABUSED CHILD

Children recently assaulted, and their families, have special needs and require separate consideration.

The protection of the child can often be ensured without prosecution of the offending adult. The desire for retribution must not be allowed to overcome the needs of the child. If criminal proceedings are taken, a probation order with the requirement of treatment is often more satisfactory for the future wellbeing of the family.

The man is likely to already have difficulties in interpreting touching in a non-sexual way. He may view children as pawns to be used for his own gratification, or include sexual abuse in a general violent response to those who should be nearest and dearest. Such a man is not helped by imprisonment in solitary confinement, or with others of similar tendencies. Warders and other prisoners regard such offenders as the 'lowest form of life' and subject them to verbal and physical abuse. Imprisonment tends to harden their attitudes and make it more difficult for them to relate to people they regard as weaker and inferior to themselves. The only justification for prison is to remove the offender from society because the facilities for treatment do not exist and there is no other way to contain their activities.

Where abuse is associated with poor parenting, modification of behaviour patterns may be possible. This is usually undertaken by social workers, a clinical psychologist, or a child psychiatrist. Anger management programmes have been described as of use, especially where the abuser has acted impulsively without control and is motivated to change. (Nicol, 1989).

Groups for older children may be used, and play therapy for younger children. Self-help groups are sometimes available, especially in association with rape crisis centres. All groups need careful supervision and in-put from experienced workers together with advice from child psychiatrists.

Mental illness in a parent is rarely a significant factor in child sexual abuse, but where this occurs a referral to an adult psychiatrist may be required.

Family approaches need to be used with caution. Children in families in which abuse has occurred are fearful and mistrustful. The use of a conjoint therapy where the abuser and victim are seen together may be harmful. In a family systems framework, individual actions, including abuse of a child by an adult, are seen as being part of the overall functioning of the family. Families do not exist in isolation and it is possible for an abusive family to engage the attention of large numbers of professionals without changing the relationships within the family. The power differential between the adult perpetrator and the abused child may be lost in the examination of the functioning of the family. The detailed analysis of repetitive, interactional sequences of behaviour which threaten or contain abusive episodes can imply that the child is on a level with the adult and an equally responsible participant. This implies that an infant or small child is somehow responsible for the abuse which is clearly absurd. Examination of family functioning should only be used where a specific outcome is sought, and where the less powerful can be protected.

It is unfortunate that there are few expert sources of help for offenders, and particularly for families in which abuse has occurred. The Family Unit at the Cassel Hospital, Richmond, Surrey has pioneered methods of working with these families. The hospital provided an in-patient setting in which the needs and rights of the child were paramount. A detailed understanding of the play of the child and the light it throws on inner thoughts and feelings was developed. At the same time, the parents' capacity to look after their children is supported. As trust developed more freedom and responsibility was allowed to the parents, unless the family had reached such a point of breakdown that they could not stay together as a unit (Kennedy, 1988).

THE DOCTOR'S PERSONAL AND PROFESSIONAL LIMITS

The primary care physician is unlikely to be involved in any of these activities. He or she needs to remain on the sidelines and to be perceived by those involved as a non-judgemental non-participant. Efforts by family members to enlist the support of the doctor for any one course of action, or to back one family member against another have to be resisted.

A caring but cool professional approach is not easy to sustain, for doctors have feelings too! The anger can be intense; not just the anger picked up from the patient but the doctor's own internal anger at the violation and recognition of his or her own inability to have prevented the abuse. Particularly when the family is already known to the doctor, denial is a common defence against these strong emotions. The result is that the patient, child or adult, trying to tell the doctor about the events, is not heard. Pointers which are obvious when the history is known may be ignored. The doctor of first contact cannot avoid playing a key role in the recognition of sexual abuse. In children presenting with organic disease, and particularly with unexplained physical or psychological symptoms, sexual abuse needs to be considered (Brown and Perkins, 1989). Similarly, adult patients with somatic complaints (not just gynaecological ones) should have the possibility of sexual abuse kept in mind by their doctors (Arnold *et al.*, 1990).

If doctors can recognize their own feelings about the subject, they will be better able to maintain a high index of suspicion. Anxieties about being involved in press reports, similar to those which accompanied the Cleveland enquiry, will be easier to deal with if recognized and discussed with colleagues.

Doctors are familiar with the difficulties they encounter when people with whom they work or socialize ask for help with their problems. When such a personal area as sexual abuse is involved, the difficulties are compounded. The nurse colleague who asks 'can I have a word about a personal problem?', the social acquaintance who corners the doctor at a party and reveals past sexual abuse, the teacher at the school attended by the doctor's children who asks for personal help after attending in-service training about child sexual abuse, all pose particular problems.

These friends and acquaintances are not patients; it is important for the maintenance of normal social life that they are referred to sources of help where they can be patients who have a professional relationship with the therapist. Doctors who offer to see such people as though they were patients are inevitably handicapped in their therapeutic endeavours by the social relationship.

Contact with episodes of sexual assault will be most difficult for those doctors with personal experience of such abuse. It may reveal individual problems which need to be dealt with to avoid harrowing re-experience of emotions which may have been deeply buried. As with the friends and acquaintances issue, proper professional help should be sought. Doctors with such problems should rapidly refer patients who have suffered sexual abuse to alternative sources of help to minimize their own personal distress.

The importance of sharing this difficult and sometimes distressing work with colleagues cannot be overemphasized. Further training to improve skills in this area should be sought by anyone interested in the field. Discussion with partners, or in seminar groups, or with a more experienced colleague can renew the doctor's enthusiasm to continue to see patients. Alone, the doctor may be overwhelmed.

Doctors need to learn their own limitations. There is a temptation for sensitive, caring doctors to try to carry all the burdens which are thrust upon them. Patients bring their concerns to the doctor; they need to be shared and examined but ultimately handed back to patients for resolution. Doctors cannot do this work on behalf of patients. Attempting to do so is arrogant and continues to maintain patients in a state of powerlessness; the very state they are struggling to escape. Doctors who are over-involved with the emotions of the patient become unable to see clearly the processes occurring between the patient and the doctor; they become as powerless as the patient and unable to provide the professional skills required. A tired doctor, burnt-out with response to constant emotional demands, is unable to use a consultation to discovery why the patient came, what the patient expects from the doctor, to examine the problem, make a plan of action or check that the patient and doctor have the same view of the situation.

Time for renewal of energy, time for normal social interactions, time for personal intimate relationships, time to do things other than the usual work, all these are part of the maintenance that a doctor must practice in order to remain emotionally healthy and of use to patients.

In a report of a day conference for child and adolescent psychiatrists and forensic psychiatrists (Bull. R. College of Psychiatrists, 1989), many of those attending said things like 'I don't want anyone to know I'm here or I will get swamped with referrals' and 'It's as if I want to find out but I'm afraid they are going to tell me'.

General practitioners do not have any choice of who comes to see them, or the type of consultation. Whoever comes through the door has to be seen and the problem heard and sorted out. General practitioners must know how to cope with the problem of sexual abuse and must be aware of the possibility in covert presentations.

MORE INFORMATION NEEDED

The field of sexual abuse is still relatively unresearched. Recognition of abuse tends only to occur in its most florid forms and the general incidence is unknown. When looked for, it is always more common than previously thought.

Further knowledge about the course and outcome both in the abuser and in the victim will enable more rational management in the future. For instance, it is suspected that abused boys may go on to become abusive adults – but the evidence is anecdotal or deduced from the information available about physical abuse of children and might be untrue for the majority.

Information also needs to be gathered as to whether abused girls tend to marry potential abusers. The low self-esteem of abused girls may favour the establishment of patterns of behaviour within the family that prevent the children, or the mother, complaining about or refusing to accept violation.

The evidence so far suggests that the outcome is worse if abuse starts at an early age, and is influenced by the duration and frequency. If the abuse is accompanied by violence rather than tenderness, and within an otherwise unsupportive family environment, the victim usually appears more damaged. However, there are patients who appear to have been extensively affected by what seems to the listener to be a fairly trivial episode, whereas others remain unscathed despite a horrific upbringing. More understanding of how these events are dealt with by individuals needs to be gained.

PREVENTION

Programmes aimed at prevention have only recently been instituted and cannot yet be evaluated. Greater awareness that the home is the commonest place for sexual violence to occur and the knowledge that almost all abusers are not mentally ill, (nor do they have diminished responsibility) helps potential victims recognize the dangers.

Teaching children at school about the boundaries of permitted touching can help. They need to know that they have a right to control access to their bodies, that certain ways of being touched are unacceptable and that they should trust their own feelings as to what they find acceptable. They need to be able to say 'no' and be given the opportunity to tell an adult if they think they have been touched in an unacceptable way. They must be heard if they do tell an adult that they feel uncomfortable about how they are being touched.

Doctors have an important role to play, not only by being available to listen and by hearing both the overt and the covert complaint, but also in acknowledging children's rights over their own bodies. Assuming that the parent can give permission for a child to be examined perpetuates the loss of autonomy: the older the child, the more important it is to acknowledge the child's own rights. Agreement should be obtained from both parent and child, unless time or circumstances prevent this. Where the examination involves an area of the body not normally touched by others, an explanation (appropriate to the age) must be made to the child of why it is necessary and the reasons given as to why it is acceptable in these circumstances (for example, the touching being done for medical reasons and in the presence of a parent or nurse).

Doctors can also help families where parenting skills are poor or when the parents have inappropriate expectations of their children. Greater awareness of the needs of children and what they require for satisfactory physical and emotional development would enable parents to improve their skills.

THE WAY FORWARD?

However, children cannot be protected against sexual violence from their parents, or women against rape, by State employees or professional workers alone. Doctors, health visitors, social workers, the police or probation officers only see a fraction of the problem and usually at too late a stage for preventive measures to be of use.

As we edge forward, the most important changes are likely to come through changes in the way children and women are viewed by society. No human being should be used by another violently or for selfish sexual gratification. The objective should be respect for individuals, adults or children, honouring their right to determine for themselves how their bodies should be used. As this Utopia is unattainable, those in primary care must maintain awareness of the possibility of sexual abuse and violence.

Sexual assault arouses very strong emotions such as disgust, excitement, anger and a desire for retribution, which may become overwhelming and prevent professionals from working effectively. Pre-existing attitudes of apostolic fervour, religious or social (including excessive feminism), may be manifested by an urge to convert everyone to the cause of diagnosing abuse to the detriment of the child. In contrast, an attitude that is too authoritarian or cynical may fail the distressed complainant. Over-identification with the victim will also prevent a doctor from working with the family or patient. But doctors in primary care cannot avoid involvement with sexual abuse. They need to examine their own attitudes and skills in order to do the work as effectively as possible.

As well as awakening within the doctor a strong wish for reparation and healing, this field is a significant intellectual challenge, presenting fascinating medical diagnostic issues and major ethical dilemmas.

REFERENCES

Arnold, R. P., Rogers, D. and Cook, D. A. G. (1990) Medical problems of adults who were sexually abused in childhood. *Br. Med. J.*, **300**, 705–8.

Brown, R. M. A. and Perkins, M. J. (1989) Child sexual abuse presenting as organic disease. *Br. Med. J.*, **299**, 614–5.

Bull. R. College Psychiatrists (1989) Child Sexual Abuse in practice after Cleveland. *Bull. R. College Psychiatrists*, **13**, 204.

Hooper, P. D. (1990) Psychological sequelae of sexual abuse in childhood, *Br. J. General Practice*, **40**, 29–31.

Kennedy, R. (1988) The treatment of child abuse in an in-patient setting, *Bull. R. College of Psychiatrists*, **12**, 361–6.

Nicol, A. R. (1989) Role of the Child Psychiatry Team, in ABC of Child Abuse. *Br. Med. J.*, **299**, 451–2.

Peebles, J., Draper, K., Sage, C., and Hutchinson, F. (1988) Sexual Abuse. *Proceedings Inst. Psychosexual Medicine*, Leicester, pp. 99–117 (limited publication).

Index